Reviews of HELPING YOURSELF WITH N

"Willard's explanation of why herbs fight disease based on their vital energy' makes for fascinating reading....offers a comprehensive overview of individual ailments and their herbal treatments. Readers interested in alternative therapies will want to investigate this volume."

---The American Library Association's "Booklist" Magazine

"As a serious and enjoyable introduction to the subject, this book shows the reader that in spite of any existing stigma, herbs are a sensible alternative for treating illness."

---"Small Press" Magazine

"When my patients ask for a book to keep at home, I recommend **HELPING YOURSELF WITH NATURAL REMEDIES.** Vitamins, minerals and herbs are all laid out according to the way they are used. The recommendations allow people in any area to find effective natural remedies."

---Dale Richards, Master Herbalist, Kamloops, British Columbia

"When first studying the natural health field, you are facing a mountain of information. The first step is to learn the simple principles of natural healing that go a long way to helping people stay healthy. **HELPING YOURSELF WITH NATURAL REMEDIES** was my guide in those difficult first months. I really appreciated the careful coverage of vitamins and minerals and the fact that the recommended herbs were easily available. Now the book is filled with my own notes and becomes more useful as time passes."

---Flo Lavallie, Saskatoon, Saskatchewan

"As a supplement retailer, getting accurate information out to the public is a great challenge. People really enjoy the informal style of **HELPING YOURSELF WITH NATURAL REMEDIES.** There is space for them to add their own notes and an encyclopedia format which makes looking things up a breeze."

---Stewart Brown, Owner of Supplements Plus, Toronto, Ontario

"The average health food store shouldn't be without a basic book which provides general and useful recommendations for health problems. **HELPING YOURSELF WITH NATURAL REMEDIES** provides good solid advice, is easy to use, and customers often end up purchasing a copy for their own bookshelf."

---Deborah Burkhart, Manager of Vitamin Warehouse, Calgary, Alberta

HELPING YOURSELF WITH NATURAL REMEDIES

Terry Willard, Ph.D.

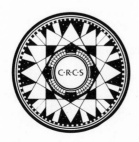

CRCS PUBLICATIONS
Post Office Box 1460
Sebastopol, California 95472
U.S.A.

Library of Congress Cataloging-in-Publication Data

Willard, Terry, 1951-
    Helping yourself with natural remedies.

    Includes index.
    1. Herbs--Therapeutic use. 2. Medicine--Formulae,
receipts, prescriptions. 3. Therapeutics, Physiological.
I. Title.
RM666.H33W55 1986   615'.321   86-9714
ISBN 0-916360-34-2

New American Edition © 1986 by Terry Willard
Originally published in Canada © 1984 Wild Rose College of Natural Healing Ltd.

INTERNATIONAL STANDARD BOOK NUMBER: 0-916360-34-2

Published simultaneously in the United States and Canada by:
CRCS Publications
Distributed in the United States and Internationally by:
CRCS Publications
(Write for current list of worldwide distributors.)

NOTE FOR HEALTH CENTERS, PRACTITIONERS & HEALTH PRODUCT DEALERS: Quantity discounts are available on this book. Please write direct to CRCS Publications for information, stating the quantity desired.

Dedication

This book is, first of all, dedicated to my lovely wife Dorothy who stands by me, gives me support and puts up with my busy lecture schedule, and to my kids Yarrow and Aiyana, whose beaming faces bring me joy!

Second, I would like to dedicate this book to the Deva of Wild Rose for pushing and helping my staff and myself in giving service to those needing it, sick or well!

Third, I would like to make a dedication to all of the patients that have given me the knowledge to write this book. Without your comments and feedback, I would not have learned so much with such practical value.

Acknowledgements

A complete list of acknowledgements would be impossible. It would include all the lecturers I have heard, all books I have read, people I meet in my day-to-day-life and, most of all, the patients I have seen in the past.

A list of people working solely on this book will have to suffice:

Illana Holloway, for suggesting the book and prodding me on.
Don Hobsbawn, editing, arranging and paste ups.
Penny Hess/Skylark, word processing, editing, and patience.
Marie Gagnon, word processing.
Dr. Ross Skaken, foreword.
Henry Garand, editing.
Steve Burger, technical editing.
Dot Willard for encouragement and time to work on this book.
Rose Danby, for editing diagrams and artwork.
Blaine Andrusek, cover photography.
Donna Shannon, editing and promotion.
James McCormick, last-minute editing and production.

Second Printing: Donna Shannon and James McCormick.

To everyone, my thanks for their dedication to the successful completion of this project!

FOREWORD

As one becomes familiar with the philosophy of health and healing, two principles emerge which dominate the basic biological functions of the human organism in health and disease.

The first is that the health or harmony of body, mind and soul are so closely interrelated that it is rare that any treatment of lasting value considers only the treatment of one of these aspects, without giving some attention to the other two.

The second premise is that for every human ill there are remedies to be found in nature, present in the fruit, herbs, seeds and creatures on this earth.

More and more we are learning that this first concept of man is an entity that functions on several interrelated levels of being. The second premise, which invites an exploration of natural healing methods, is the subject of this book.

Hippocrates, the father of modern medicine, stated: "Let your food be your medicine, let your medicine be your food.".

When we examine the preconditions, principal factors and forces which create, sustain and evolve life on our planet, we find them to be: atmosphere (air), hydrosphere (water), cosmosphere (solar and other cosmic radiations whose nature we do not yet fully know), lithosphere (the earth's crust with its chemical elements) and the botanosphere (steppes with the grasses, the different seed-bearing plants, the forests and trees, especially trees with fruits). These are the factors, the forces, the preconditions of the appearance of the evolution and of the maintenance of life. We have a heredity which scientists call "ontogenetic experience" in the organism. These factors have a very important hereditary influence on our organism.

Our Twentieth Century technology is able to harness these energies in their natural state as well as their products and processes in tablets, tinctures, fluid extracts, special preparations that concentrate by pre-infusing (quadgyric method) and potentizing (homeopathic method).

The author has had more than a decade of Clinical application and experience in the use of these energies in the form of vitamins, minerals and herbs. He lectures to health professionals as well as to the public throughout Canada, the United States and Europe.

I am confident you will find this book of great value in your life and the lives of your family.

Dr. Ross Skaken, B.A., N.D., F.A.C.A.C.N.

Author's Note

Please Note: The information in this book is presented as a matter of general interest only. It is not in any way a prescription for any specific person or condition. It consists of the best information available to the author through his research of the scientific literature and personal observation. Other research and observation may produce differing information and opinions. In every case, where a specific health problem or concern exists, competent professional advice should be sought.

TABLE OF CONTENTS

Introduction

Did you ever notice on a bus, at a party or at your place of work that most people don't have a smile on their faces? Did you ever notice in yourself or others around you that by the end of the work day you really don't have that much energy left to do some of those personal or family things you really would like to do? A lot of people are walking around only partly "energized" as there seems to be something continuously draining them. Well, that is what this book is about: trying to use some simple methods to make you healthy enough to feel good at the end of the day!

In looking at some of the most common ailments encountered by the average family, you will be presented with natural remedies that have helped people over the centuries as well as some of the most current research information. These remedies are generally without side effects (except where noted) and, as is explained in the section "Herbal Philosophy", they support the body with energy instead of "stealing" it.

By using these methods, combined with some personal observation and adjustment, we can work on our bodies in a natural way and perhaps gain that extra "plus": feeling good!

In writing this book I've tried to keep it as simple as possible by using easy-to-understand language and easily obtainable herbs, herbal formulas and supplements.

It should be remembered at all times that you have to deal with a person as a whole individual, not just as separate parts. We seldom have just one little thing wrong with us. We are a complex mixture of mental, emotional, spiritual and physical attributes, and as such, everything has to be considered. The physical body alone is a very complex mechanism; for example, you can't have a liver problem without it affecting the rest of the body. The blood will not be cleansed properly, the kidneys and skin will be burdened by the elimination of toxins, and the digestive system will suffer from lack of proper bile production.

Consider this writing as an information base and use it as a guideline only, as it is not meant to replace the Health Practitioner. It should not be used as a self-prescribing book. The information is set out to help you understand how the various herbs can work, especially in complex herbal formulas where one herb's interaction with the next expands the quality of the whole so as to be much more than the sum of the individual parts (Synergy). Herbs are one of the most important forms of medicine and food, having a long history as tested cures. Even today, in the Twentieth Century, more people world wide are being treated daily with herbs than with any other modality of medicine. This is something we often forget, living on our isolated continent of North America.

It should be understood that herbs work synergistically with vitamins, minerals and other therapeutic modalities and are usually more effective when used together.

Let's go on to the practical aspects of this workbook!

HOW TO USE THIS BOOK

This book is set up in five sections:
1. Herbal Philosophy: understanding the energy of herbs.
2. Herbal and Synergistic Formulas.
3. Encyclopedia of Ailments and Treatments.
4. Appendices.
5. Cross-reference index.

The first section of the book gives the reader an understanding of herbs, their energy, and their differences from pharmaceuticals. The serious student may want to study it, as it deals with the essence of why herbs should be used, along with some guidelines for choosing and preparing them.

The second section deals with many of the formulas found in the enclyclopedic section. These are the formulas that I prefer and use regularly in my practice. Some I have formulated myself, and some have been formulated by other herbalists (both modern and traditional). Most of the formulas are in a marketable form, meaning that they should be easily obtainable in your local Health Food Store or through a Health Practitioner.

The formula section should be continually cross-referenced to the encyclopedic section for determining the best formulas and dosages to be used in the various situations.

The third and largest section of the book is the encycolpedia of ailments. This should be used as a reference and is most effective when cross-referenced with the formulas section and appendices. Each reference is in several parts:
1. Description of the problem.
2. Recommended actions.
3. Single Herbs useful for the ailment.
4. Herbal Formulas that can be used.
5. Synergistic Vitamins and Minerals.

For some ailments I have also included suggested progams to follow and/or brief case studies.

Section four is one of the appendices covering diets, exercises and other procedures generally used throughout the encyclopedic section, including a glossary of terms you might not be familiar with.

Section five of the book is the index used to locate items not easily found in the encyclopedic section.

The encyclopedic order of the main body is for simplicity. The book was written in a workbook format with plenty of space for annotations. Use this space well and in future years I think you will find it very beneficial.

THE PHILOSOPHY OF HERBAL USE

The most important issue in herbal use is why are they different? What is it that sets herbs apart from any other healing agent? To the herbalist, herbs are unique because they are not just a group of chemicals. Each herb has its own nature which, for want of better word, we call its personality. The concept of herbal personality is the basis of herbology and has played a major role in herb use for thousands of years.

Most of the world's people continue to use herbs as their primary form of medication. While various cultures may not have our knowledge of biochemistry of plants or the same perspective on the structure of the human body, all herb using cultures have an appreciation for the 'personality' of herbs. A herb is a living substance and has its own constellation of energy. We don't think of ourselves or our pet dog as being merely a conglomeration of physical parts. We have emotions, mental concepts and spiritual feelings. It would be silly to assume that herbs don't have patterns of energy beyond mere molecules. North American Indians believe that the spirit of the herb is directly involved in a battle with an illness when herbal healing takes place. Other cultures (e.g. the Chinese and East Indian) choose their herbs by taste, smell and colour along with energies related to fire, metal, water, wood and earth – features which we might not think were important for healing. A first step in understanding herbology lies in appreciating the fact that we should focus just as much on the essence or 'personality' of the herb as on the scientific descriptions.

ALTERNATIVE PERSPECTIVES IN MEDICAL THEORY

Healing methods around the world take many approaches. The western medical philosophy we are most familiar with (medical doctors and allopathy) has generally taken a mechanical-scientific view towards health. If you have a broken arm, it can be splinted. If there is a missing chemical in a biochemical pathway, they can replace it or make a suitable piece to fit in. If a bacteria or virus is present in your body, a powerful biochemical means can be found to destroy it or subdue it. One must admit that western medical professionals are good mechanics who have helped many people, who have tackled disease in powerful ways and can give us everything from artificial hearts to trauma care.

In our own past and around the world an alternative means of organizing medical care is known. This system starts with theories of life energy and relates it to the physical forms of human beings and diseases they have. Medicine in the traditions of European herbology, American Indian medicine, East Indian medicine and Chinese medicine is seen as the conscious manipulation of energy for healing the human body.

This energy is known by many names: the life force, chi, prana and also VITAL ENERGY. Vital energy is the term which modern herbologists use because it is the purpose of non-allopathic medicine to keep this energy flowing correctly through the body or, if the flow is improper, to return it to its natural path. The Herbalist feels that disease is caused by stagnant or incorrectly directed energy due to some energy blockage. The herbalist's role is not so much to attack a disease, but to maintain the natural flow of vital energy. The energy itself will rid the body of disease.

A CLOSER LOOK AT VITAL ENERGY

Vital Energy is the flow of energy through one's body. This can be likened to a river that gets unnaturally clogged or dammed, stopping the normal flow of its energy. The river forms a stagnant pool which, as I'm sure you've all seen, breeds abundant algae and insects in a swampy condition.

There are two very different ways to get rid of such things as mosquito larvae, abundant algae and other undesirables:

1. The way I was told in high school to get rid of mosquito larvae was to pour oil on the water so they couldn't breathe. You can also dump poisons into the water to make the environment unbearable for these organisms. Of course this also destroys most other life-supporting functions in the pond.

2. The other way is to work on dislodging the obstruction damming the river. This lets the river flow and clean itself naturally.

Our bodies are quite similar to this river. Disease is the blocking of the natural vital energy that flows through our body. Let us say that at least some of these energy streams are the acupuncture lines in the body. When the energy is flowing properly along these pathways, it naturally keeps the body clean, just as the river does. Like a river, the bodily energy flow can handle a certain amount of waste.

To fight disease in our bodies, we can dump in all kinds of chemicals to make the environment unliveable for the intruder. We can, as an alternative, unplug the system and get the energy flowing again. As in the case of rivers, if these energy pathways are not obstructed and no wastes are put into them, the job of cleaning is not as taxing and the energy can then be used to support life.

Thus, our job is not to try to kill disease in our bodies. Our job is to keep the body free of energy obstruction so the natural vital energy flows throughout the body selecting, disintegrating, absorbing, assimilating and converting foodstuffs. In other words, we don't try to take on the role of trying to cure diseases; we merely assist the vital energy in our bodies to flow in an unobstructed way.

Herbs, in this sense, are not really considered medicines. They are just specialized foods which help vital energy flow, being somewhat selective in where their energy is directed. The 'personality' of the herb will be attracted to certain areas of the body similar to different types of people associating in 'like-minded' groups. For example, Juniper Berries have a 'personality' that strongly influences the kidneys.

This "Vital Energy" is just one part of a modern herbalist's understanding of how herbs work. To understand the chemical interactions the herbs have on the human physiological mechanism is just as significant. Most herbalists feel that one is fairly ineffective without the other. The "Vital Energy" of the herb is what makes it work. For something to work in a live biological system it has to have life energy. Herbs, with their own life essence, work in harmony with the biological system to enact healing.

A pharmaceutical will copy the chemical makeup of a herb, but it can only work by overpowering the system, 'stealing' some of the body's life energy (as it has none of its own). Pharmaceuticals are usually used when the body needs this life energy the most. In a medical crisis, for example, the pharmaceutical's power and fast action of the chemical are necessary. Of course, there may arise some side effects that have to be dealt with, but usually they can be best balanced out by herbal treatment later.

For the everyday non - crisis health problems, herbals have a long proven history of cure. After all, most of the herbals we are dealing with have been tested on millions of people over thousands of years. Their methods of use have been very thoroughly studied.

The Ecology of Energy

The ecology of the energy that we use in our body, and for that matter, any biological system, is important to understand. We don't **really** eat because it tastes good or because it looks nice! The main reason for eating is to take energy into our body. All the food we eat is really little packets of energy that we use to animate ourselves, think or even read this page. We are a big nutritional factory that processes foodstuffs to give us energy, at least on the biological level. I eat an apple because it looks good, tastes good but more specifically because I need the energy it gives me. This energy is the Vital or biological energy that is in the food. Where does this energy come from?

The major energy source of our solar system is the sun, of course, and that is where our energy originates. Some 93 million miles away, the sun acts as a very efficient nuclear reactor, and produces untold amounts of energy. The planet Earth is fortunate in that it has developed a system for capturing this solar energy. In Fig. 1.1 (Page 6) we have a summary of the whole process.

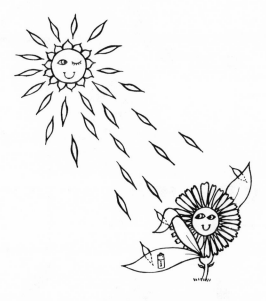

Fig. 1·2

The Sun shines upon our planet where plants have the capability of capturing some of this energy, thus putting the energy into the biological system (Fig 1.2). Plants are the only biological system that can capture this solar energy to be used by the rest of the biological systems on this planet. One can easily see that the plant kingdom has a very important responsibility in being the sole collector of biological energy for our planet. It is also easy to see that the plant kingdom takes this responsibility very seriously, as plants seem completely dedicated to their job and the sun! If I have a potted plant in my window it will bend towards the sun. If I turn the plant around it will switch its direction again orienting itself toward the sun. Of course it is impossible for us to consider what a plant might feel, but this level of complete dedication to the sun that the plants give almost seems like they 'feel' that the sun is their God. Could this be why some ancient human cultures conceived of the Sun as **their** God?

THE ECOLOGY OF ENERGY

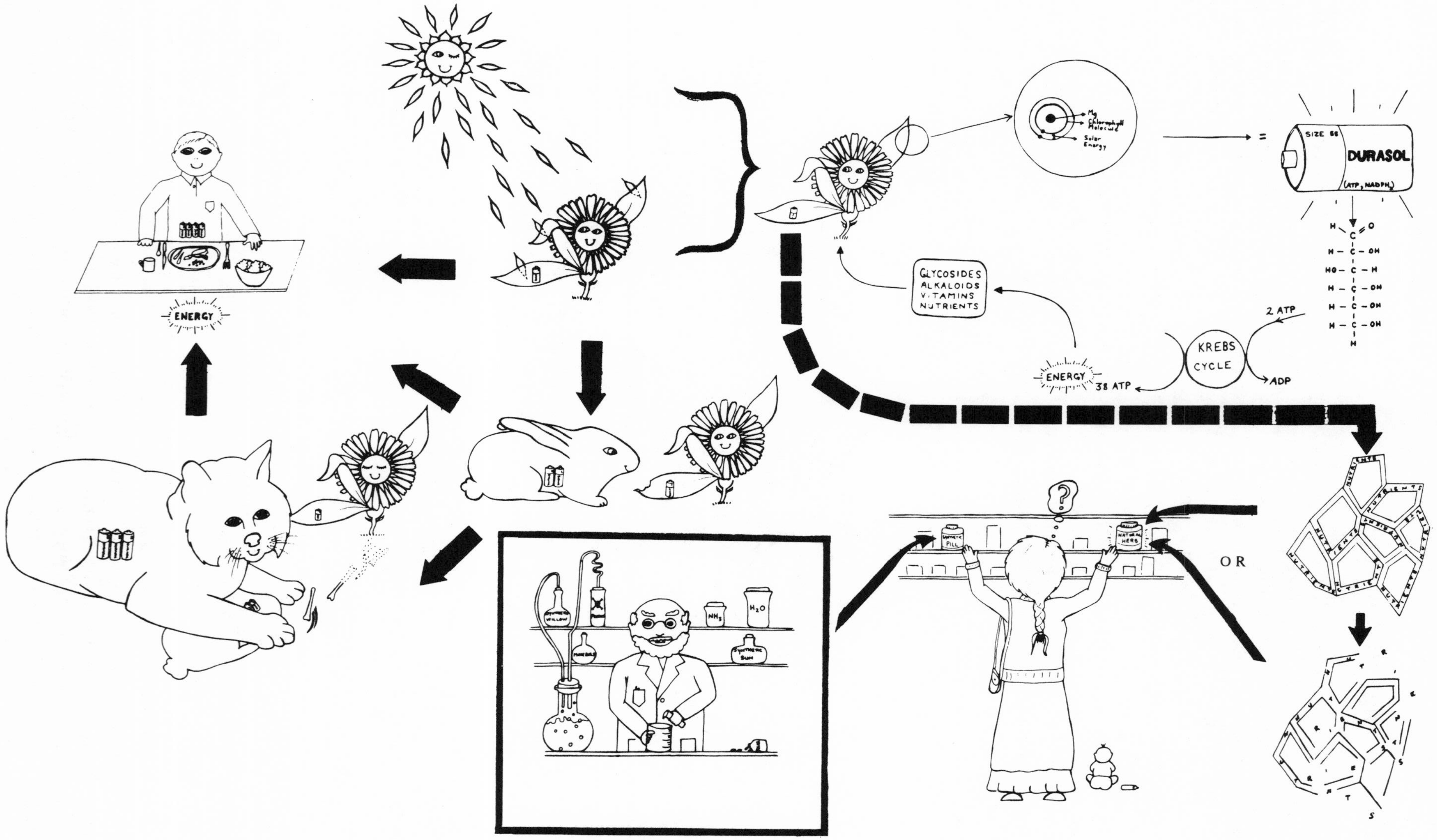

Fig. 1·1

Looking at the situation a bit closer we can see what happens on a molecular level (Fig 1.3). When the Solar energy hits a chlorophyll molecule in the green parts of the plant the Magnesium (Mg) atoms' electrons are excited. In our simplified diagram of the Magnesium atom (Fig 1.3 & 1.4) we see that the orbital of the electron has expanded. We could make this anology to a person jumping for joy when something very exciting is happening. The plant in its complete dedication to the Sun seems to get very excited (or at least its Mg molecules do!) when the radiation of the Sun shines upon it. This whole process is very simplified but is of the utmost importance, because this excitation of Magnesium represents the entrance of solar energy into the Earth's biological system. All other organisms live off this energy. Can we say then that the primary source of biological energy on our planet is the dedication that the plants have to the Sun? (Some Alchemists believe that this is a good model to look at. If complete dedication is given to one's God, then all the energy necessary for existence will be given back.)

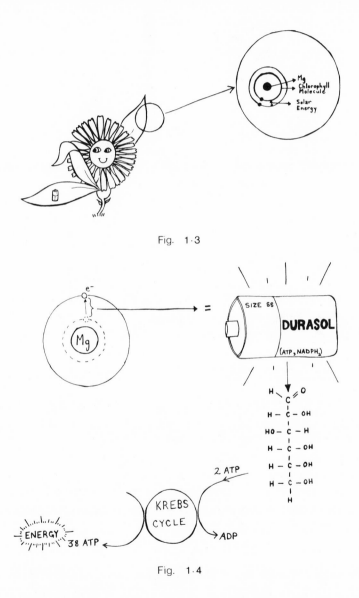

Fig. 1·3

Fig. 1·4

This 'excited' energy is passed onto other molecules, such as ATP and NADPH2, for short - time storage in the plant cell (Fig 1.4). We can consider them solar batteries, and in my diagram I have signified them as a "Durasol Solar Battery" (the solar-topped battery). This Solar energy, now converted to Biological energy is available to do work in the organism or to be stored in the form of nutrients such as a simple sugar called glucose. The basic energy manufacturing process of nature occurs through a series of chemical reactions, one of the best being "the Krebs Cycle". If we now take two units of working energy and put it into the Krebs Cycle, with this basic stored energy, we get 38 units of working energy out on the other side of the reaction! This energy can be used elsewhere to make raw chemicals into various nutrients for the plant such as Glycosides, Alkaloids, Vitamins and many other nutrients. The key point here is that it takes the excited energy of the original solar energy, being passed along the system, to activate these molecules. All of these biologically made nutrients have their molecules made up of excited electrons, energy from the original solar excitement of the Magnesium molecule. Chemicals are basically shells that carry energy. We survive on biological energy. I have to eat living organisms with biological energy to survive. If this were not true my lower jaw would be different, being more like a bulldozer for scooping up dirt, thus getting all of the minerals needed for my body. The plants do this for me; they pull the minerals out of the ground, filling them with live biological energy so that I can use them. Since my primary need for eating is to obtain this biological energy, I eat plants or organisms that eat plants.

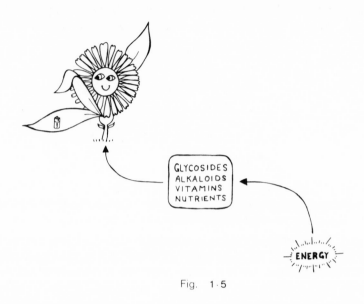

Fig. 1·5

To gain its energy a herbivore eats plants and a carnivore eats herbivores. (Fig 1.6 & 1.7) To get our energy we can eat from any of these groups, as we are of a higher group. (Fig 1.8) It is interesting to note that any waste materials, either in the form of excrement or parts not completely eaten, are recycled via the micro-organisms. This compost makes it very much easier on the plants because now they do not have to convert all nutrients into biologically usable forms, since some nutrients absorbed from the soil are already in this form, and only need to get charged up.

Now what does all of this have to do with feeling good with natural remedies?

It is easy to see that to keep our solar batteries charged we need biological energy. What is most dis-ease, but a lack of proper biological energy? When I am sick I need certain types of nutrients to help heal me. These nutrients are really chemicals that are shells specific to my energy needs. Since I am looking more for the energy contained in the chemical than the shell itself I want the chemical with the best type of energy available, biological energy. I will normally be better served with chemicals that come from the biological realm.

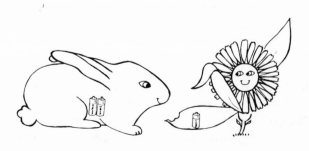

Fig. 1·6

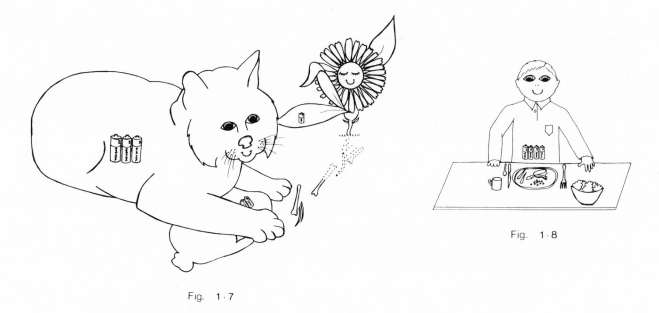

Fig. 1·7

Fig. 1·8

Along comes Man (Fig 1.9) with his isolated views of the universe and looks at the problem to make a "better" way. Looking at the way a plant makes a chemical that has traditionally been used for a certain health problem, man realizes he can make it cheaper and faster, therefore making profits for himself and his company. The big problem is that the scientist didn't realize that there is much more to plants and man than just chemicals. Man cannot live by chemicals alone. The only way that these chemicals can work in a biological system is to be activated by biological energy. Synthetic chemicals have to take the energy from the biological system they are in. These synthetic chemicals, which might be useful in crisis medicine, don't really have a place in our day to day life.

These synthetic chemicals, because of their lack of Biological energy, have to be taken in fairly large quantities to work. Synthetic chemicals work like a bulldozer pushing chemicals down certain biochemical pathways. Since there are often side branches to these pathways a person often gets side effects from them. Herbs, on the other hand, have the Biological energy already in them, so the same quantity of chemical is not needed to achieve the job. This has a threefold benefit:

1. Because the biological energy in the herb is in "harmony" with the biological needs of the body the herbal chemical most often goes down the right pathway without side effects.

2. We don't have the possibilities of as many side effects because of the lower quantity of chemical.

3. Biological energy is **given** to the body during this process, not **taken** as in the case of the synthetic chemical.

These benefits are not without any drawbacks though. Herbal energy takes much longer to form its benefit. Herbals are just not as fast as synthetic chemicals. This is why a smart Herbalist will often surrender to a practitioner of synthetic chemicals in a crisis situation and then will try to clean up the side effects later.

A consumer (Fig 1.10) has to make aware decisions of how to best help themselves and their family in disease situations; to be able to decide between the synthetic way and the natural way. That is what this book is about - Feeling Good with Natural Remedies.

There is still another major question to answer about herbs and that is: In what form is it best to take herbs?

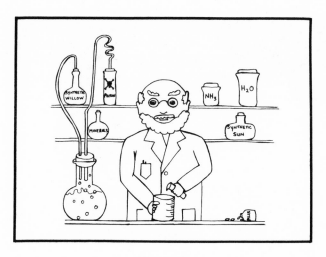

Fig. 1·9

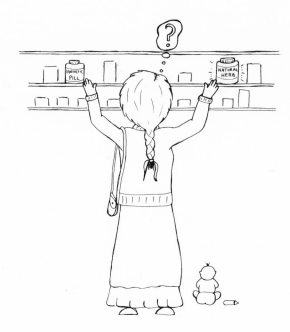

Fig. 1·10

METHOD OF HERBAL PREPARATION

The essence of a herb can be best obtained in the usable form of a menstruum. The most common menstruums are water, alcohol and apper cider vinegar.

Different common methods for the preparation of Herbs

Herbs have traditionally been available in four forms: teas (infusions), capsules/tablets, fluid extracts and tinctures. Each form has its own advantage. Teas are valuable because the medicinal ingredients of the herb are in solution (menstruum), thereby allowing efficient absorption of the active ingredients. Capsules, on the other hand, are very convenient. They can be taken anytime and anywhere, and because the herb is encapsulated, its often unpalatable taste is shielded. Fluid extracts and tinctures are valuable because they are the most potent form of the herb. They also store for long periods of time, and because of their strength, small doses are as effective as larger doses of the same herb in another form.

However, each of these forms has its disadvantages. Medicinal teas are often unpalatable and inconvenient, requiring special preparation; therefore, people do not take them as often as they should. Capsulated crude herbs, in spite of their remarkable convenience, are hard to digest because the active ingredients of the herb are entrapped within cellulose cages with no menstruum to release the essence. Only an optimally functioning digestive system (something we seldom see) can fully release them. Fluid extracts and tinctures taste, in a word, terrible and are messy. If they are not handled with caution, stained clothes are often the result. Also, with teas, fluid extracts, and tinctures, part of the herb and, consequently, part of its value is missing. As in the making of a tea, we leave the bag and drink the tea, tinctures and fluid extracts throw away the bulk herb after extraction.

The Quadgyric Method

The QUADGYRIC METHOD is special. It combines all the advantages of the above four forms and yet eliminates all of their disadvantages. By PRE-INFUSING the herbs in special solutions (menstruums) in an advanced manufacturing technique, it liberates the active ingredients of the herbs from their cellulose entrapment. They are then redeposited on their original cellulose base. This is similar to making a tea but keeping the base that was used in the first place. You get the whole herb and nothing but the herb, with its essence activated.

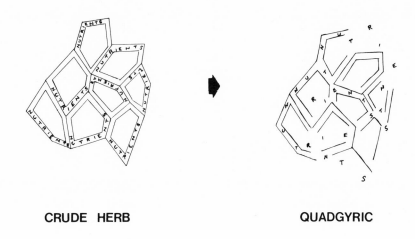

CRUDE HERB   QUADGYRIC

WHY THE QUADGYRIC METHOD IS SUPERIOR

1. THE ACTIVE INGREDIENTS ARE IN A READILY ABSORBABLE FORM.
2. THE VALUE OF THE ENTIRE HERB IS RETAINED.
3. THE ESSENCE OF THE HERB IS IN AN ACTIVATED FORM BECAUSE IT WAS RELEASED BY A MENSTRUUM.
4. IT IS PALATABLE.
5. IT IS CONVENIENT.

In the following section I have listed the formulas that are available in quadgyric form.

HERBAL AND SYNERGISTIC FORMULAS

THE RATIONALE OF DESIGNING A HERB FORMULA

Introduction

Creating a herbal formula is analogous to bringing together a group of people and forming an inter-working, cooperative, and harmonious whole. If each member of the group has an overbearing and truculent nature, each would try to force his point of view on the others. The result? Little would be accomplished because there would be no spirit of cooperative interaction. The point, then, is that in preparing herbal formulas, a systematic approach is far more conducive to revitalizing the mind and body. Remember, that is a very important point.

RELY ON PROVEN FORMULAS

The first thing to remember when dealing with herbal formulas is that many already on the market or in books have been tested through time and have been used successfully for decades, centuries or even a thousand years. There is nothing at all wrong with relying on formulas that have withstood the test of time and proven themselves in the process.

When you do prepare your own formulas, the following rules are important to consider:

1. Three parts of the formula should consist of the herb(s) actively working to correct the specific disorder.

2. One part of the formula should be soothing (demulcent) to the impaired tissue.

3. One part should be nourishing and strengthening.

4. One part should have eliminative properties.

5. One part should be concerned with proper nerve supply (if needed).

6. One part should be stimulating (if needed).

When devising a herbal formula, never take a "shotgun" approach. A formula consisting of a large number of herbs is seldom as effective as one consisting of a fewer number - the formula simply becomes "too confusing" and its effectiveness is lost!

EXAMPLE

Let's assume that you wish to prepare a good general formula for the kidneys:

RULE #1 states that you should have three parts of the formula made up of a herb(s) which is a specific for correcting the particular disorder.

So, what we need to do is to take three parts of one or more herbs which have their specific influence on the kidney functioning; because we are preparing a "general" formula, we will allow ourselves to choose three individual herbs, namely:

1 Part	Uva-Ursi
1 Part	Juniper Berries
1 Part	Buchu

RULE #2 states that one part of the formula should be soothing to the improperly functioning or damaged tissue.

This part of the formula serves to "smooth out the rough edges" of the other herbs. Since our kidney formula will induce the elimination of concentrated urine and possibly calculi, stones or gravel, we would incorporate, as an effective demulcent:

> 1 Part   Marshmallow Root

RULE #3 states that one part of the formula should be nourishing and strengthening.

This component of the formula is often made up of the same herb(s) that we employ in applying Rule #1 (their concentration becomes increased). In this particular example, though, we will employ another herb, specifically:

> 1 Part   Parsley leaves

RULE #4 states that one part of the formula should have eliminative action.

This component of the herb is needed to help remove the byproducts that result from building, toning, and strengthening the impaired area and/or to eliminate excess morbid and useless material present in the affected area. (ie. To eliminate excessive and morbid mucus in the digestive tract.)

In preparing our formula, we will want to eliminate calculi, gravel, and stones by slowly dissolving them. Our indicated herb is therefore:

> 1 Part   Gravel Root

RULE #5 states that one part of the formula should enhance nerve supply to the affected area (if needed).

In this case none is desired!

RULE #6 states that one part of the formula should be a stimulant (if needed).

Ginger will satisfy this, although we do not want too much stimulant, just good blood circulation. In applying this Rule, we try to increase supply to the specific area, both to bring in the needed nutritive material of the herbs and also to help eliminate toxic material.

Our formula, then, is now complete and consists of:

Equal Parts: Uva-Ursi
Juniper Berries
Buchu Leaves
Marshmallow Root
Parsley Leaves
Gravel Root
Ginger Root

After this procedure the formula must be employed clinically. After testing this formula for one year we found that too many people, approximately 3%, were dropping kidney stones too fast and too large, so gravel root was eliminated for a wider public appeal. Five years later the results are still very satisfactory.

HERBAL AND NUTRITIONAL FORMULAS

The following formulas are listed generically. Your health practitioner or health food store can help you find the herbs or products you need.

ARTHRITIS FORMULA

A Quadgyric Formula

This herbal formula aids the body with arthritis or rheumatism by stopping swelling and inflammation and easing the pain in muscles and joints. While acting to reduce pain, it also aids in eliminating underlying toxins and metabolic problems that create arthritis. This formula has also been found useful in weight control.

Devil's Claw and Yucca are the most important herbal ingredients in Arthritis formula, both having a saponin-type chemical which acts similarly to cortisone. These chemicals seem to either stimulate the adrenal glands to produce cortisone or in some way work as a precursor to it. In the herbal form they have been shown to markedly reduce inflammation while reportedly dissolving calcium deposits.

Red Clover and Chaparral are both excellent alteratives, aiding in cleansing the system of excess toxicity and acidity, often an underlying cause of arthritic-related problems.

Valerian is an excellent nervine and is used to ease the pain associated with these problems.

SUGGESTED DOSAGE: Two to four tablets, twice to four times a day depending on degree of problem. It is strongly suggested to follow an alkaline forming diet. (See Appendix)

Contains: Devil's Claw, *Harpagophytum procumbens*
Yucca, *Yucca sp*
Chaparral, *Larrea divaricata*
Red Clover Blossoms, *Trifolium pratense*
Valerian root, *Valeriana officinalis*

B AND B TINCTURE

B and B tincture is a Dr J. R. Christopher formula. It is used mostly as an antispasmodic. It has been successfully employed for all kind of spasms, including spastic colons, muscle spasm, hiccups and even used in cases of epilepsy.

SUGGESTED DOSAGE: 3 - 10 drops as needed, usually three times daily.

Contains: Black Cohosh, *Cimicifuga racemosa*
Blue Cohosh, *Caulophyllum thalictroides*
Blue Vervain, *Verbena hastata*
Scullcap, *Scutellaria lateriflora*
Lobelia, *Lobelia inflata*
alcohol tincture with glycerine

B-HERB

B-Herb is a natural ratio vitamin B-complex supplement. It contains all of the B vitamins including "B-15" Calcium Pangamate. This supplement also has 500 mg. of vitamin C and is prepared on a herbal base.

Because B-Herb contains Niacin, the natural form of B-3, rather than Niacinamide as its B-3 source; it can produce a harmless transitory flush after use. This flush is useful in persons with poor peripheral circulation.

Niacin has also been used to lower blood cholesterol and in the treatment of alcoholism and schizophrenia. Niacin has been a key nutrient in the development of 'mega-vitamin' therapies.

SUGGESTED DOSAGE: Two tablets daily after a meal or as recommended by your Health Practitioner.

CAUTION: Keep out of reach of childern. Niacin may in certain persons cause a transient but harmless flushing of the skin.

Contains:	
Thiamine Mononitrate	25 mg
Riboflavin	13 mg
Pyriodoxine HCl	34 mg
Niacin	120 mg
Vitamin B12	45 mcg
Folic Acid	3 mg
d-Pantothenic Acid (d-Calcium Pantothenate)	100 mg
Para - Aminobenzoic Acid (PABA)	24 mg
Choline Bitartrate	100 mg
Inositol	5 mg
d-Biotin	64 mcg
Vitamin C (Ascorbic Acid)	500 mg

Other Ingredients:
Calcium Pangamate (N,N-Dimethylglycine and Calcium Gluconate)   10 mg
Alfalfa, Rosehips, Rice Bran and Passion Flower

BONE FLESH AND CARTILAGE

This is one of Dr J.R. Christopher's most famous formulas. To sum up this formula in a word, it is 'magical'. If anything is wrong with your bones, flesh or cartilage, this formula is of use. Use it on sprains, torn ligaments, bruises, breaks and a multitude of other connective tissue needs. It is also beneficial to take this same formula internally while applying it externally.

Fomentation

For a fomentation take the above formula and make into a strong tea (1 tablespoon herbs to 1 cup boiled water and steep 20 minutes). Strain the tea and soak a piece of natural fiber material, such as cotton, in the tea. Lightly wring out the cloth and wrap it around the affected area. Cover with a plastic bag and then a towel. Apply twice daily for an hour if possible.

This formula also comes in the form of an ointment. Though more convenient, it is not quite as effective but certainly does the job.

Taking this formula internally either in a tea or a capsule form will really aid in the action of the fomentation.

Contains: Oak Bark, *Quercus muhlenbergii*
Marshmallow Root, *Althaea officinalis*
Mullein Herb, *Verbascum thapsus*
Wormwood, *Artemisia absinthium*
Lobelia, *Lobelia inflata*
Scullcap, *Scutellaria lateriflora*
Comfrey Root, *Symphytum officinale*
Walnut Bark (or Leaves), *Juglans sp.*
Gravel Root, *Eupatorium purpureum*

CALCIUM/MAGNESIUM
PLUS
VITAMIN D

Calcium/Magnesium plus D is not "just another" simple calcium tablet. This specially balanced formula has a Calcium/Magnesium ratio of 2:1 as recommended by most leading nutritionists. Calcium lactate is used in this formula because it has been found to be one of the most easily assimilated forms of calcium, particularly in the presence of adequate Vitamin D supply.

Supplemental calcium intake may be an important factor in preventing the development of osteoporosis (loss of bone minerals, usually in old age).

Magnesium Oxide is one of the most easily assimilated forms of magnesium. Absorbtion is further aided in this formula by bromelain.

Kelp and Rose Hip Extracts are included to supply a large variety of multi mineral and 'mystery' factors, such as bioflavonoids, that aid in the utilization of calcium/magnesium metabolism.

SUGGESTED DOSAGE: Three or four tablets daily, or as recommended by your Health Practitioner.

Contains:

Calcium (Calcium Lactate)	150 mg
Magnesium (Magnesium Oxide)	75 mg
Vitamin D	100 IU
Bromelain	20 mg
Kelp	50 mg
Rose Hips Extract	10 mg

C-HERB 500

This 500 mg. Vitamin C on a herbal base is a supplement complete with the factors occurring with it in nature.

Necessary for many of the body's cleansing processes, Vitamin C is recognized as an antioxidant, detoxifier and an essential nutrient for the formation and maintenance of connective tissue (teeth, gums, bone, muscle and cartilage). It is speculated that it is necessary for the release of folic acid from food and that it facilitates the absorbtion of iron.

Rutin and Hesperidin Complex have often, along with the Bioflavonoids, been called Vitamin P or "permeability factors", decreasing the 'leakiness' and the fragility of capillaries. Many nutritionists think of this combination as a vitamin C complex as they are all contained in foods high in C and seem to act in similar ways within the body. *The Complete Book of Vitamins* (Rodale Press, 1977) states that of these, the citrus bioflavonoids are the most potent.

Rose Hip Powder is included to ensure that any of Nature's "mystery" factors are also present in this food. The herbal base in this tablet is added for the same reasons.

SUGGESTED DOSAGE: One tablet daily, or as recommended by your Health Practitioner.

Contains:

Vitamin C (Ascorbic Acid)	500 mg.
OTHER INGREDIENTS:	
Lemon Bioflavonoids	250 mg.
Hesperidin Complex	50 mg.
Rutin	50 mg.
Rose Hip Powder	250 mg.
Parsley, Red Raspberry and Mullein Leaves	

CLEANSING FORMULA

A Quadgyric Formula

The key actions of Cleansing formula are cleansing the bloodstream, muscle and lymphatic system tissue of toxic waste material and metabolic by-products, and delivering these wastes out of the body via the urinary system. It has been used by many as an adjunct to fasting and other cleansing programs.

Red Clover and Chaparral are two of the strongest herbal alteratives known, and have been used successfully in many cases of cancer, heavy metal toxicity, lymphatic toxicity and mucus congestions.

Mullein and Marshmallow both work on the lymphatic system, soothing the mucus membranes specifically, while working as a demulcent throughout the whole system.

Uva-Ursi and Parsley are diuretics which aid in collecting and eliminating excess body fluids through the urinary tract.

Burdock is an effective alterative, hepatic and tonic. Echinacea is alterative, diaphoretic and tonic.

SUGGESTED DOSAGE: One tablet a day for the first week, increase by one tablet per day each week, until six tablets (2-3 times daily) are taken by the sixth week. This dosage is normally continued for six months.

Contains: Red Clover blossoms, *Trifolium pratense*
Burdock root, *Arctium lappa*
Echinacea leaves, *Echinacea angustifolium*
Chaparral leaves, *Larrea divaricata*
Mullein leaves, *Verbascum thapsus*
Uva-Ursi leaves, *Arctostaphylos Uva-Ursi*
Parsley leaves, *Petroselinum sativum*
Marshmallow root, *Althaea officinalis*
Cascara Sagrada, *Rhamnus purshiana*

DIGEST

DIGEST is a capsulated formula of digestive enzymes and HCl (Hydrochloric Acid) that aids in digesting food. The capsule ensures that the various digestive aids can be specially prepared to be released in their proper environment: i.e. HCl (hydrochloric acid) in the stomach, and pancreatin in the duodenum.

Glutamic Acid HCl and Betaine HCl are two forms of hydrochloric acid that are properly buffered to aid in increasing stomach acidity for the first stages of protein digestion. Not only is HCl important for protein digestion, it is necessary to stimulate both hormone and digestive enzymes required in other digestive functions further down the digestive tract. Calcium Ascorbate is a salt form of vitamin C that is also an excellent buffer for HCl in the stomach.

Pancreatin NF is a combination of pancreatin enzymes amylase, lipase and protease which are prepared so as not to be released until they reach the duodenum. These digestive enzymes aid in hydrolyzing fats, digesting proteins and converting starch.

Bromelain and Papain are added for their well known function of aiding digestion while stimulating the digestive system to produce its own digestive enzymes.

SUGGESTED DOSAGE: One or more capsules in the middle of the two major meals of the day or as directed by a Health Practitioner.

Contains: Glutamic Acid HCl   100 mg.
Betaine HCl   100 mg.
Calcium Ascorbate   50 mg.
Pancreatin   360 mg.
Bromelain   80 mg.
Papain   75 mg.

FEMALE FORMULA

A Quadgyric Formula

Designed for women, this is used to correct hormonal imbalances such as those that occur at puberty, after pregnancy, menopause, upon the cessation of birth control pill usage or after a hysterectomy. This formula has also been found to be very useful for alleviating discomfort due to menstrual cramps, also reducing edema and depressions associated with the menstrual cycle. It may also strengthen the female organs.

Female formula has also been used in hormone upsets in men, especially effective in the first stages of hormone related balding.

Dong Quai, a major Chinese herb for thousands of years, is by far the most important herb in this formula. This herb is often considered 'female ginseng' as it builds up the female organs and regulates hormones the way ginseng does in males. Black Cohosh and Blessed Thistle are all emmenogogues used both to build up and regulate the female reproductive system. Cramp Bark's specific function is to reduce cramping in the female organs.

SUGGESTED DOSAGE: Two tablets, three times daily.

Contains: Dong Quai, *Angelica sinensis*
Black Cohosh, *Cimicifuga racemosa*
Blue Cohosh, *Caulophyllum thalictroides*
Blessed Thistle, *Centaurea benedicta*
Cramp Bark, *Viburnum opulus*

FIG SYRUP

Fig syrup can be obtained in most health food stores or can easily be made yourself.

Take: Two Cups of Figs (Mission are the best)
Four Cups of Water

Soak the figs overnight, and in the morning add more water until the volume of the water is approximately twice that of the enlarged figs. Put in a non-aluminum double boiler and simmer for 20 minutes. Strain and Refrigerate.

SUGGESTED DOSAGE: One to two tablespoons, twice daily.

GLUCOSE FORMULA

A Quadgyric Formula

Designed to enhance carbohydrate metabolism, Glucose formula equalizes sugar levels in both high and low blood sugar conditions. It has also been found useful to help the hypoglycemic handle stress. In addition to its sugar regulation function, it is formulated to strengthen the pancreas and adrenal glands while giving assistance to pancreatic digestive enzymes, making it a general pancreatic tonic.

Cedar Berry has been shown to be very successful in regulating insulin production, thus controlling sugar metabolism to a great extent.

Uva-Ursi works as an effective diuretic and is used for adrenal support.

Licorice root also gives adrenal support and aids in regulating blood sugar levels.

Mullein is useful for dealing with low-grade infections in the pancreas and aids in all glandular function.

Cayenne stimulates circulation, aiding in delivering the nutrients to the pancreas.

SUGGESTED DOSAGE: Two tablets, three times daily.
In cases of diabetes this product should be used under the supervision of a qualified Health Practitioner.

Contains: Cedar Berries, *Juniperus monospernum*
Uva-Ursi, *Arctostaphylos uva-ursi*
Licorice root, *Glycyrrhiza glabra*
Mullein leaves, *Verbascum thapsus*
Cayenne Pepper, *Capsicum minimum*

GREEN LIFE

Green Life is a famous formula of V.E. Iron. and is generally used as a gastrointestinal detoxifier and oxygenator. The high nutrient quality of this product along with its bulking factor make this an excellent remedy to use during fasting, in winter months when fresh vegetables aren't as available or just as a general building - detoxifier.

SUGGESTED DOSAGE: 4 - 12 tablets, two to six times daily.

Contains: Dried extracted juices of one or more young growing Cereal Grains:
oats
wheat
corn
barley
rye

Plus:
                                        Papain
                                        Beets
                                        Seaweed
                                        Vitamin C

HERBAL SLEEPING TABLETS

This formula comes in a tablet form and is a very good herbal relaxant, pain reliever and sleeping tablet.

For sleeping we usually suggest 2 - 6 tablets a half hour before bed. For pain up to 6 tablets six times daily.

Contains: Valerian Root   dessicated extract
            Passion Flower   "
            Hops (female flowers)   "
            St. Johns Wort   "
            Balm Leaves   "
            Hawthorn (leaves & flower)   "
            East Indian Valerian   "
            Chamomile   "
            Hops glands (lupulin)   "
            Vitamin B1
            Soya Lecithin

LIVER FORMULA

A Quadgyric Formula

Liver formula is used to stimulate bile flow, decreasing Cholesterol buildup in the gallbladder while dissolving calculi. This herbal formula can be used to detoxify the liver (hepatic) area, strengthen liver functions for blood cleansing and aid nutrient storage and many general hepatic functions.

Black Radish is the major ingredient and can lower blood bilirubins levels through its cleansing actions on the liver. Black Radish has also been shown to be the best herb for dealing with gallbladder congestion.

Barberry root bark, which has been used since the time of Galen and Dioscorides, is very successful for stimulating bile flow and for detoxification of the liver. Grieve in *A Modern Herbal* says that it is an ". . . excellent remedy for functional derangement of the liver."

Parsley root and Dandelion root are both known for their hepatic qualities and for the ability to dissolve gallstones or prevent formation.

Wood Betony is a soothing hepatic which also strengthens the spleen, thereby giving additional blood cleansing and supporting liver function.

SUGGESTED DOSAGE: One to two tablets, twice to four times daily.

Contains: Black Radish, *Raphanum sativus nigra*
Barberry root bark, *Berberis vulgaris*
Ginger root, *Zingiber officinale*
Marshmallow root, *Althaea officinalis*
Parsley root, *Petroselinum sativum*
Wood Betony, *Pedicularis canadensis*
Cramp Bark, *Viburnum opulus*
Dandelion root, *Taraxacum officinale*

LOWER BOWEL TONIC

A Quadgyric Formula

Lower Bowel Tonic comes from a generic group of herbal formulas that are specific for the colon and benefit the digestive tract. The **exact** ratio of herbs has great significance on how well it works.

Although it has a cleansing or 'laxative' effect, its major functions are to increase muscle tone and flexibility of the intestinal wall and to correct neural and hormonal control throughout the system. Many practitioners of natural methods strongly believe that a clean and healthy colon is the first and maybe the most important step toward better health. The problem is that many 'laxative type' formulas are 'addictive' in the sense that the longer you take them the more you need to take to get the same action. **This formula is quite different.** Working on muscle tone, it **strengthens** the colon, instead of just causing bowel movement. After taking this formula for several months the patient needs less for the same action.

Cascara Sagrada, Buckthorn and Turkey Rhubarb are the major components as all have a group of glycosides in them that stimulate catharsis. Two of these glycosides, emodin and chrysophanic acid, work similarly to the brakes and gas pedal in a car, controlling the motility of the colon. This control causes the major building feature of this formula. Cascara Sagrada not only acts as a laxative but restores natural tone to the colon.

Ginger and Fennel seeds aid in reducing griping or nausea in the intestinal tract during the cleansing phase. Golden Seal strengthens the mucus membranes while Raspberry leaves work as a demulcent soothing the intestinal tract. Barberry aids in cleansing the liver at the same time producing bile, which stimuates catharsis. Lobelia works on nervous control and the Cayenne increases the blood circulation.

SUGGESTED DOSAGE: Two tablets three times daily or as needed.
Diarrhea is often experienced for the first few days. If this continues after the third day, decrease dose accordingly.

Contains: Cascara Sagrada, *Rhamnus purshiana*
Buckthorn, *Rhamnus frangula*
Ginger root, *Zingiber sp*
Barberry, *Berberis vulgaris*
Golden Seal root, *Hydrastis canadensis*
Raspberry leaves, *Rubus idaeus*
Fennel seed, *Anethum foeniculum*
Turkey Rhubarb, *Rheum palmatum*
Lobelia, *Lobelia inflata*
Cayenne pepper, *Capsicum minimum*

LUNG FORMULA

A Quadgyric Formula

This herbal formula is specific for dilating bronchial tubes while cleansing mucus from the bronchials, lungs and sinuses. It has been found useful for airbound allergies, sinus congestion and lung problems.

Ma Hueng, the major ingredient of this herbal formula, has been for over 5,000 years one of the most important herbs of Chinese medicine. Its major chemical, ephedrine, used extensively in Western medicine since 1923, works on the autonomic nervous system to cause dilation of the bronchial tubes and alveoli. It has also been shown to be a great cleanser of the respiratory mucus membranes.

Mullein leaves (demulcent, expectorant and diuretic), and Coltsfoot leaves (expectorant, demulcent and diuretic) are both specific for the respiratory system.

Golden Seal is considered the 'King of the mucus membranes' aiding in **building** the quality, while **regulating** the quantity of mucus in the respiratory system. Lobelia herb works on the nerve supply to the lungs and is also an excellent expectorant.

Cayenne stimulates blood circulation, aiding in the supply of nutrients. It has been called the purest and most certain stimulant in the herbal materia medica.

SUGGESTED DOSAGE: One to two tablets, two to three times daily.

Should be used only under the supervision of a qualified Health Practitioner in cases of high blood pressure or heart disease.

Contains: Ma Hueng herb, *Ephedra sinica*
Mullein leaves, *Verbascum thapsus*
Golden Seal root, *Hydrastis canadensis*
Coltsfoot leaves, *Tussilago farfara*
Comfrey leaves, *Symphytum officinale*
Marshmallow root, *Althaea officinalis*
Lobelia, *Lobelia inflata*
Cayenne pepper, *Capsicum minimum*

MELBROSIA MALE

FLOWER POLLENS	98%
Ascorbic Acid	2%

MELBROSIA FEMALE

FLOWER POLLENS	93%
Royal Jelly	5%
Ascorbic Acid	2%

Both these formulas have had fairly strict studies conducted in Europe showing that well over 50% of the men and women taking the respective formula become more fertile.

It has been shown to increase both sperm count and sexual desire in men.

SUGGESTED DOSAGE: One to two capsules twice daily. For women it is best to open the capsule just using the contents. For men take the whole capsule.

PSYLLAX

This formula is a bulk laxative and hydrophillic bulking agent that soothes the intestinal tract. It is specific for colon irritations, ulcerations and spasms. As a bulking agent it has functioned to suppress appetite while cleansing the intestinal tract, making it very useful for weight control programs. It is also an effective astringent in firming up diarrhea. The major factor in determining if it is used as a laxative or an astringent is the amount of liquid taken during the day. Taking less than 3 - 4 cups of liquid will give Psyllax a firming action, over 7 cups gives it a laxative action.

Psyllium husk, the major component of this formula causes the bulking action in a mucillagenous base.

Comfrey, Whey powder, Marshmallow and Slippery Elm all work on the quantity and quality of mucus in the intestinal tract.

Echinacea herb, Shepherd's Purse, Bayberry and Bentonite all aid in detoxification.

Wild Yam works on spasms and cramping in the intestinal tract.

SUGGESTED DOSAGE: One tablespoon in a glass of water or juice (tastes best in tomato or apple) morning and evening, or as directed by a practitioner.

Contains: Psyllium Husk, *Plantago psyllium*
Comfrey, *Symphytum officinale*
Whey powder
Marshmallow root, *Althaea officinalis*
Slippery Elm bark, *Ulmus fulva*
Echinacea herb, *Echinaceae angustifolia*
Powdered Bentonite
Shepherd's Purse, *Capsella bursa*
Wild Yam, *Dioscorea sp.*
Kelp, *Fucus versicuosus*
Bayberry bark, *Myrica cerifera*

MUSCLE RELAXANT

A Quadgyric Formula

The key ingredient in this formula is Kava Kava root, the most powerful herbal muscle relaxant known. Working on the motor units (the point of muscle-nerve coordination), Kava Kava increases general flexibility, aiding in soft tissue tension and helping in structural adjustment.

Capsicum, the most effective herbal circulatory stimulant, increases blood flow to speed healing of injured tissues.

Cramp Bark is specific for cramping of all kinds.

Ginger combines antispasmodic and stimulant characteristics to carry the active ingredients to the afflicted area.

Lobelia and Lady Slipper Root are powerful nervines and antispasmodics which reduce pain and alleviate tension due to over-exertion of injuries.

Red Clover blossoms help to clean impurities from the blood and tissues while acting as a light stimulant and antispasmodic.

SUGGESTED DOSAGE: Two tablets, three times daily, increase as needed.

Contains: Kava Kava, *Piper methysticum.*
Cramp Bark, *Viburnum opulus*
Cayenne Pepper, *Capsicum minimum*
Ginger Root, *Zingiber sp*
Lobelia, *Lobelia inflata*
Lady Slipper Root, *Cypripedium acuale*
Red Clover, *Trifolium pratense*

NERVE FORMULA

A Quadgyric Formula

Nervousness in individuals varies with their ability to cope with circumstances and surroundings. It could be described as a state of restlessness, mental or bodily, or both.

Symptoms could be that the person is fidgety and easily startled, sleepless, restless, anxious or fatigued. A feeling of unpleasantness or sometimes even of fright can occur making concentration difficult to impossible.

Valerian yields isovalerianic acid giving a soothing, calming and sedative effect. Mistletoe yields viscin, Scullcap yields scutellarin, Hops yields lupulinic acid and humulon, and Lady Slipper Root yields a volatile oil, all giving a soothing and calming effect.

SUGGESTED DOSAGE: One tablet before meals and one at bedtime (4 daily)

Contains: Valerian, *Valeriana officinalis*
Mistletoe, *Viscum album*
Scullcap, *Scutellaria lateriflora*
Hops, *Humulus lupulus*
Lady Slipper Root, *Cypripedium acuale*
Passion Flower, *Passiflora incarnata*

TIBET 28

It is likely that the complex pharmacological content of Tibet 28 involves numerous mechanisms acting simultaneously to achieve its remarkable healing properties. A few contributing mechanisms have been suggested:

Two studies indicate that platelet aggregation threshold is increased by this product. Two more studies indicate that it alters immunological responses.

An analysis of its constituents suggests that the formula helps normalize arterial wall interaction with the blood. An analysis of the range of indications suggests that it influences the levels of prostaglandins. Several researchers are currently investigating these hypotheses.

Tibet 28 is used for: Angina Pectoris, Peripheral Arterial Occlusion, disabilities of old age and poor circulation. It has been clinically tested in Europe for the past 15 years and is proven highly effective for treating cardiovascular disorders. In Switzerland it is licensed by the I.K.S. (the Swiss equivalent of the "Food and Drug") and is currently one of the best-selling remedies for circulatory problems, especially atherosclerosis. Tibet 28 is used as a sole therapeutic agent or as an adjunct to other therapies such as chelation, dietary modification, nutritional supplementation, and standard pharmaceutical and surgical intervention. According to reports from several physicians, it has helped restore normal functions of the cardiovascular system in a large number of patients.

SUGGESTED DOSAGE: Two - twice daily (1/2 hour before meals)

Contains: Spiral flag, *Costus amarus*
Iceland moss, *Cetraria islandica*
China berry, *Melia toosendan*
Myrobalans, *Terminalia chebuba*
Cardamon, *Elettaria cardamomum*
Red Saunders, *Santalum rubra*
Sorrel, *Amomum medium*
Camphor, *Cinnamomum camphora*
Gypsum, *Gypsum fibrosum*
Hardy Orange, *Poncirus trifoliata*
Columbine, *Aguilegia veridi*
Licorice, *Glycyrrhiza uralensis*
Ribwort, *Plantago lancolata*
Knotgrass, *Polygonum aviculare*
Golden cinquefoil, *Pontentilla aurea*
Cloves, *Syzygium aromaticum*
Gingerlily, *Hedychium spicatum*
Heartleaved sida, *Sida cordifolia*
Lettuce, *Lactuca sativa*
Valerian, *Valeriana officinalis*
Marigold, *Calendula officinalis*
Aconite, *Aconitum sp.*
Binder, 85 mg. glucose

CHINESE STOMACH FORMULA "PO CHAI"

"Po Chai" is a famous Chinese formula. I know Practitioners who claim that this formula has basically saved their lives. It may not have really saved their lives, but it certainly helped. Chinese herbalists recommend "Po Chai" after a big feast when you know you have eaten too much. It reputedly relieves gas and indigestion often accompanying big meals. "Po Chai" is traditionally used for diarrhea, stomach upset, overindulgence of alcohol, and also all gastro-intestinal problems.

SUGGESTED DOSAGE: one or two vials with some hot tea.

Contains: Saussurea L.C
Halloysite
Chrysanthemum M.R.
Oryza Sativa L.
Mentha H.B.
Trichosanthes K.M.
Poria Cocos Wolf
Artrctylodes L.
Pueraria L.
Pogostemon C.B.
Angelica A.L.
Magnolia Off. Rehd. Et. T.

C.Tangerina H. Et. T.
Sun Kook
Coix L. - Jobi L.

RENAL FORMULA
(KIDNEY-BLADDER FORMULA)

A Quadgyric Formula

Renal Formula is formulated to cleanse and build the renal (kidney/bladder) system. It has also been found useful for clearing congestion in the prostate gland.

Uva-Ursi contains a chemical called arbutin which changes into the urinary antiseptic hydroquinone in the kidneys, thus aiding to rid the urinary tract of infection. Uva-Ursi is also an excellent diuretic, cleansing the kidneys and bladder, and is considered excellent in dissolving kidney sediment such as sand, gravel and even stones.

Juniper berry is a urinary antiseptic as well as a diuretic.

Buchu is specifically for the prostate and is an excellent diuretic.

Parsley, a mild and soothing diuretic, is one of our most nutritious herbs, being exceptionally high in Vitamins A and C.

Marshmallow is a very useful demulcent for the urinary tract, soothing the mucus membranes so as to avoid irritation from concentrated urine or calculi deposits.

Ginger is used to stimulate peripheral circulation and to avoid griping in the urinary tract.

SUGGESTED DOSAGE: One or two tablets, two or three times a day.

*** As Uva-Ursi is most effective in an alkaline urine, it is suggested that an alkaline diet be followed when using this herbal formula.

Contains: Uva-Ursi, *Arctostaphylos uva-ursi*
Juniper Berries, *Juniperus communis*
Buchu leaves, *Barosma crenata*
Parsley leaves, *Petroselinum sativum*
Marshmallow root, *Althaea officinalis*
Ginger root, *Zingiber sp*

STOMACH FORMULA

A Quadgyric Formula

Stomach Formula is designed to not only work as a general tonic for the stomach and digestive system, its major purpose is to stimulate the production of hydrochloric acid (HCl). Found very beneficial for the stimulation of other digestive enzymes from the pancreas and liver, it is an advantage to a large proportion of North American society which does not digest food properly. Many herbal practitioners use this formula at the beginning of any rebuilding program when lack of proper digestion might be a factor in the overall condition of the patient.

Meadow Sweet (Spirea) is the major herb as it has been shown to regulate gastric secretion, **increasing HCl** in hypoacidic conditions and **decreasing** it in hyperacidic conditions of the stomach.

Golden Seal is considered the 'King of the mucus membranes', its specific action being a tonic to the digestive system.

Fennel and Fenugreek both work as cleansing agents, working on excessive mucus in the digestive tract and as digestive tonics. Fennel also acts as a carminative, reducing griping of the intestines and relieving indigestion. Fenugreek is a demulcent and is soothing for inflamed conditions of the stomach.

Cayenne increases the circulation to the parietal cells of the stomach thus ensuring that the proper nutrients are present for the manufacture of HCl.

Lobelia aids in both autonomic nerve and hormone control so that higher level controls will be in place to co-ordinate and regulate the digestive functions. This formula, instead of giving the body digestive enzymes as an outside aid, stimulates the body to produce its own.

SUGGESTED DOSAGE: One to two tablets with the two major meals of the day.

NOTE: If a person has a large accumulation of mucus in the digestive tract, some nausea may be experienced during the first few days of use. This happens with less than 10% of users and may be avoided by taking the supplement in the middle of the meal.

Contains: Meadow Sweet, *Spiraea ulmaria*
Golden Seal root, *Hydrastis canadensis*
Lobelia herb, *Lobelia inflata*
Fennel seed, *Anethum foeniculum*
Fenugreek, *Trigonella foenum*
Cayenne pepper, *Capsicum minimum*

SUPER DAY

Super Day is a complete mega vitamin/mineral formula. Probably the main reason Super Day has become so popular is due to the fact this formula doesn't have the combination of the antagonistic supplements of Iron and Vitamin E in the same formula. It has been long known by nutritionists that if iron and Vitamin E are ingested within 4 hours of each other they bind to each other making it impossible for either to be absorbed into the blood stream. Some nutritionists go a bit further and feel that large consumption of these two supplements together over a long period of time can cause a drying action in the intestinal villi and thereby inhibit the absorption of other nutrients.

This complete formula has all the essential vitamin and minerals including 10 B vitamins.

SUGGESTED DOSAGE: One tablet daily or as recommended by a nutritionally oriented Health Practitioner.

Contains:	Vitamin A	10,000 IU
	Vitamin D	400 IU
	Vitamin C	250 mg.
	Thiamine	10 mg.
	Riboflavin	10 mg.
	Niacinamide	100 mg.
	Pyridoxine	10 mg.
	B 12	15 mg.
	Folic Acid	5 mg.
	d-Biotin	10 mg.
	Pantothenic Acid	10 mg.
	Choline	50 mg.
	Inositol	10 mg.
	Iron	10 mg.
	Calcium	125 mg.
	Magnesium	50 mg.
	Zinc	1.5 mg.
	Iodine	.15 mg.
	Potassium	15 mg.
	Copper	1 mg.
Other Ingredients:	Lemon Bioflavonoids	30 mg.
	Rutin	30 mg.

ENCYCLOPEDIA
OF AILMENTS
AND TREATMENTS

ABSCESS

An abscess may occur anywhere in the body and is a condition indicating local infection. White blood cells, known as leukocytes, collect in pockets in the infected area together with dead tissue cells and other substances to form pus - a dense opaque fluid. The function of the white blood cells is to fight infection and assist in rebuilding damaged tissue.

Recommended Action

Initially, a good drawing poultice made up of a combination of the 'single herbs' should be spread thickly over the entire area to bring the abscess to a head. Hot onions or fresh ground garlic (applied after a coating of olive oil), hot pumpkin or hot uncooked tomatoes can be used in lieu of the suggested herbs if they are unavailable. After expansion, bursting and drainage is complete, a good healing and tissue building poultice should be applied. The herbs may also be taken internally to speed healing, and at the same time a ten-day cleansing diet should be implemented. Removing mucus-forming foods from the diet and thoroughly cleansing the blood should prevent a recurrence of the condition.

Single Herbs: Hops (drawing); Comfrey (heals and rebuilds tissue); Garlic (disinfectant and tissue builder, apply a layer of olive oil first to prevent blistering); Chaparral, Burdock root or Echinacea (blood cleansers); Golden Seal root (disinfectant), Slippery Elm bark (soother and builder).

Combinations: A good drawing poultice can be made from 3 parts Golden Seal root, 2 parts Myrrh, 2 parts Slippery Elm bark, 1 part Hops and 1 part Comfrey. This poultice should be alternated with the fresh ground Garlic poultice mentioned above. For the necessary internal cleansing, take two capsules of cleansing formula, twice daily after meals. The bowel must be kept clean through use of Lower Bowel Tonic if necessary.

Synergistic Vitamins and Minerals: Vitamin C 500 mg., three to six times daily; Vitamin A 10,000 IU, two times daily. Apply Vitamin E oil after abscess is drained.

ACNE

Acne, a chronic disorder of the sebaceous glands which produces oily substances on the skin, occurs most commonly during puberty and adolescence. At this time, sex-related hormones are especially active and affect the secretions of the sebaceous glands. Hormonal imbalance can be caused by emotional stress resulting in excessive oil secretion. When the system attempts to excrete toxins through the skin, it causes the oil to become dry and hard, thus clogging the pores producing swelling, soreness and redness. A common modern diet high in meat, concentrated starches and sugars loads the system with toxic waste. This diet also lacks the necessary nutrients for maintenance of an adequate hormone balance. The result: an impure bloodstream with improper hormone balance and resulting acne. Bacterial infections are often associated with acne and are the direct result of picking or squeezing which irritates the skin eruptions.

Recommended Action

A change of diet is very important, starting with a 7 - 10 day cleansing diet (see Appendix) to eliminate toxic wastes in the blood and bowels. Avoid strong acidic foods such as meats, sugars and refined starches. Whole grains help to correct hormonal imbalances and therefore should be included in the diet after the cleansing diet. They are especially useful if sprouted or soaked overnight to change their pH. Millet, buckwheat and brown rice already have a suitable pH.

Single Herbs: Burdock root, Dandelion root, Echinacea or Sassafras (blood cleansers); Kelp, Alfalfa and Dandelion root (vitamins & minerals); Buckthorn, Turkey Rhubarb, Cascara Sagrada (bowel cleansers); Liquid Chlorophyll, Siberian Ginseng, Aloe Vera.

Combinations: Lower Bowel Tonic (bowel cleanser), cleansing formula. If hormone imbalance is suspected (as in puberty or after childbirth), use Female Formula for both males and females to readjust hormones. If liver problems are suspected, use the Liver Formula.

Synergistic Vitamins and Minerals: Vitamin A, B Complex, Vitamin C, Calcium, Magnesium, Zinc, Vitamin E and Multi-Vitamins and Minerals.

Suggested Program:

Start with a 7 to 10 day cleansing diet, then adopt a maintenance diet.

Breakfast: One Liver formula (if associated with a weak liver), two Lower Bowel Tonic, Cleansing formula (start with one a day the first week; increase by one tablet per day each week until six are taken daily, two with each meal), Carotene Vitamin A 20,000 to 30,000 IU, two B Complex, Vitamin C 500 mg., Calcium 100 mg., Magnesium 50 mg., Zinc 50 mg., One Multi-Vitamins and Minerals.

Morning Snack: Vitamin C 500 mg.

Lunch: 1/4 cup Aloe Vera juice or gel.

Afternoon Snack: Vitamin C 500 mg.

Supper: Same supplements as breakfast.

Evening: B-Complex with 125 mg. Niacin

AFTERBIRTH PAINS

These spasmodic pains occur immediately after childbirth and during the next few days. Uterine contractions are experienced the strongest while nursing the baby. Their function is to prevent hemorrhage by constricting the capillaries in the uterine wall where the placenta was recently attached. The cramps serve a necessary and useful purpose, but may sometimes cause severe discomfort.

Single Herbs: Fennel (antispasmodic); St. Johns Wort (astringent and sedative); Cramp Bark (antispasmodic); Dong Quai, Siberian Ginseng.

Combinations: Female formula (aids in adjusting hormones), Nerve Formula, Herbal Sleeping Tablet; if colon is not active use Lower Bowel Tonic.

Synergistic Vitamins and Minerals: Vitamin E, B-complex, Magnesium Phosphate (6x) tissue salt, Calcium/Magnesium formula.

Suggested Program:

Two Female formula three times daily, two capsules (two parts Dong Quai, one part Cramp Bark) two times daily, 600 mg. Calcium, 300 mg. Magnesium, Magnesium Phosphate (6x) tissue salt (10 drops four to six times daily), Lower Bowel Tonic as needed.

AGUE

Ague (recurrent spasmodic shaking) is commonly associated with malarial fevers. Unlike other fits of shivering, this condition often continues after normal body temperature has been restored. As the condition progresses, feverish spells alternate with chills. The body attempts to warm itself by spontaneous contraction of the involuntary muscles. Malaria, pneumonia and some other fever-producing maladies can be accompanied by or preceded by Ague.

Recommended Action

The best treatment is to encourage the fever with Diaphoretic herbs and plenty of moist heat until it breaks, unless it approaches dangerously high levels. In this case Febrifuge herbs should be employed to reduce the fever (see Fevers).

Single Herbs: Thyme or Hops (febrifuges); Bayberry, Blessed Thistle, Catnip, Tame Sage, Chamomile, Yarrow (diaphoretics).

Synergistic Vitamins and Minerals: B-Complex, Vitamin C, Calcium, Magnesium Phosphate (6x) tissue salt.

ALLERGIES

Hayfever, asthma, hives, nausea, dizziness, diarrhea, headaches, chills and inflammation of the skin are common allergic reactions. Allergens create these conditions in persons who are hyper(over) sensitive to them. In an effort to rid itself of the obnoxious substance, the body overreacts to the presence of the allergen and produces large quantities of antibodies and excessive amounts of histamine.

Recommended Action

Oversecretion of histamines can be inhibited by using herbal antihistamines; however, one should change to a cleansing diet which is low in mucus to obtain long-term relief. Cleansing herbs are beneficial in ridding the body of any accumulated mucus and drinking steam-distilled or reverse osmosis water increases the effects of both diet and herbs. See specific conditions (sinus, respiratory, skin, etc.) for relief from these symptoms. Often many allergies disappear when the body is cleaned out. Clean lungs, with little mucus, usually stop lung allergies. Food allergies are often alleviated if the digestive system is restored to full capacity with a clean colon. Skin eruptions can be aided by cleansing the blood and colon.

Allergy Testing

There are many ways to test for allergies. The two simplest ones that you can do at home are the "Coca Pulse Test" and a Kinesiology test. I have included both of these in the Appendix section of this book.

Single Herbs: Alfalfa (nutritive and to balance hyperacidity); Ma Hueng herb (natural antihistamine and cleanser); Chaparral, Burdock Root or Comfrey (cleansers); Bee Pollen (reported to build up immunity to allergens when taken orally in very small but gradually increasing amounts); Horseradish root (a very fast - acting antihistamine); Parsley, Raspberry (eliminates mucus from the system).

Combinations: Parsley and Raspberry leaf (equal parts in a tea); Lung formula (for respiratory allergies); Stomach formula, digestive enzymes (food allergies); Lower Bowel Tonic (to keep the colon active) and Cleansing Formula.

Synergistic Vitamins and Minerals: Digestive enzymes (to aid in digestion), Vitamin A, B Complex, Vitamin C, Calcium.

AMOEBIC DYSENTERY

In this condition the intestinal tract becomes invaded by *Entamoeba histolytica*, a parasitical microorganism which is usually transmitted by contaminated foods or liquids. The symptoms include diarrhea, abdominal pain, fever, lack of appetite and general weakness, with blood and mucus being visible in the stool in severe cases. If all these symptoms are present, it means the parasites have multiplied to such an extent as to have caused abscesses, ulcers or tumors in the lower intestines. If they migrate to other organs, such as the stomach or liver, it is possible for severe complications to result. If they become encysted, they will be difficult to reach and remove. This disease is most common in areas with poor sanitation, such as the tropics, although carriers may be found virtually anywhere.

Recommended Action

The diarrhea can be relieved by use of demulcent and astringent herbs, while the parasites can be dealt with specifically by use of garlic (taken orally and/or as an enema). Even encysted amoeba will be removed by the use of garlic over a period of time.

Combinations: "Po Chai", Psyllax.

ANEMIA

There are many types of anemia, which is basically a blood disorder. All forms result in weakness, fatigue, loss of appetite, aches and pains, heart and breathing difficulties, and the characteristic paleness of anemia. Anemia is due to a lack of oxygen reaching the various body tissues. This can be caused by not enough hemoglobin (oxygen-carrying substance in the blood) or not enough erythrocytes (red blood cells). Hemolytic anemia (involving the destruction of red blood cells) can occur as an allergic response to drugs or transfused blood. Rh factor anemia and sickle-cell anemia are inherited. Aplastic anemia (insufficient or incomplete bone marrow producing red blood cells) is caused by too much x-rays, radiation treatment or drug and chemical poisoning. Iron deficiency anemia usually results from an iron-poor diet or through not digesting and absorbing iron, but may also be caused by an excessive loss of blood. A lack of certain nutritional elements, such as Vitamin B-12, B-6, folic acid or lack of HCl in the stomach, can cause anemia as they are essential to the development of red blood cells. Iron is located at the core of the hemoglobin molecule and is responsible for binding with oxygen in order to carry it throughout the body. Hemoglobin accounts for 65% of the body's iron.

Recommended Action

Adding iron to the diet, either as a supplement or through foods such as whole grains (which are rich in manganese), will benefit iron-deficient anemia. Copper and Vitamin C are required to absorb and retain iron. Vitamin B-12 is necessary in Pernicious Anemia and can be found in animal protein, fish, dairy products, sea vegetation and naturally fermented foods (sauerkraut, yogurt, miso and rejuvelac). Rejuvelac is the liquid left after soaking wheat in water (let liquid stand for four days between the temperatures of 65 and 90 degrees F.). HCl and calcium are in turn required in order to assimilate B-12.

Single Herbs: Beet powder, Yellow Dock and Alfalfa (organic iron); Comfrey (blood cleanser and cell proliferant); Dandelion root and Siberian Ginseng (blood builders); Kelp, Alfalfa, Dandelion root and Barberry root bark (vitamins and minerals).

Combinations: Cleansing formula, Liver formula, Stomach formula, Digestive enzymes (if lack of digestive enzymes is suspected).

Synergistic Vitamins and Minerals: B-Complex with B-12, B-6, Pantothenic acid, Folic acid, PABA, Vitamin E, Bone Meal, Vitamin C, Organic Iron. Also helpful are dessicated liver, beet juice, crude blackstrap molasses, sesame seed (Vitamin T factor), and digestive enzymes (promotes assimilation of iron and B-12).

Suggested Program:

Breakfast: Two Beet Powder or Yellow Dock Capsules, One Siberian Ginseng, Organic Iron (5-10 mg.), one complete B-Complex (as under Synergistic Vitamins and Minerals), Vitamin C 500 mg., Betaine Hydrochloride 500 mg. (if stomach acid is low), one tablespoon Blackstrap Molasses, one Calcium/ Magnesium plus D, one Dessicated Liver tablet.

Lunch: Vitamin C 500 mg., one Siberian Ginseng, Vitamin E 500 IU.

Supper: Same as Breakfast.

ANGINA PECTORIS

This condition, apparently feeling similar to a heart attack, lasts only a few minutes. It is characterized by chest pains that may be felt as only a mild tightness or pressure, or may be so extreme as to produce intense aching. (Sometimes, too, pain can radiate from the chest to the shoulder and down the left arm.) These pains are a result of the heart tissue not receiving enough oxygen (due to a diminished blood supply from the coronary arteries) and are often quickly relieved by rest. This is known as myocardial ischemia and is generally caused by arteriosclerosis of the coronary arteries. For a first-time sufferer the distinct resemblance to a heart attack will generally result in great anxiety. Once aware of the condition, the sufferer can easily deal with it, lessening the overall anxiety experienced.

Recommended Action

The person should immediately attempt to relax both mentally and physically. This will help put an end to the pain as the relaxed heart muscle will cause the blood vessels to dilate (open), decreasing the need for oxygen while increasing the heart's ability to pump blood and deliver oxygen. Adopting a diet low in sodium and high in potassium and adding fresh fruits and vegetables to the diet are essential for long-term relief. Muscle tone and blood vessel flexibility are improved through the use of Vitamin E and Lecithin, while the entire circulatory system is strengthened by the use of Vitamin C and natural B-complex vitamins. Potassium is absolutely essential to proper heart function. Garlic is effective both as an antiatherosclerotic, preventing buildup of deposits on the artery wall, and as a vasodilator by opening the blood vessels.

Single Herbs: Lobelia Extract (relaxant); Elderberry Extract (potassium); Hawthorn Berry tincture (heart food and strengthener); Cayenne or Cayenne Extract (circulatory tonic and antiarteriosclerotic); Garlic, Kelp.

Combinations: Nerve formula (sedative, pain reliever), Cleansing formula (cleanse blood to prevent recurrence), Tibet 28 (cleanse out circulatory system).

Synergistic Vitamins and Minerals: Vitamin A, B complex with B-12, B-15 (N,N-Dimethylglycine and Calcium Gluconate, also referred to as Calcium Pangamate), Vitamin C, Vitamin E, Potassium, Calcium/Magnesium and Lecithin.

Suggested Program:

Immediate supplements: 10 drops Lobelia Extract, 20 drops Cayenne extract, or 1/2 tsp. Cayenne pepper in water. Rest for a few days. Slowly increase exercise, such as walking and swimming. Adopt a diet low in sodium and high in potassium with an emphasis on whole grains, fruits, vegetables and a liberal use of Garlic. No red meat and limited fish, fowl and dairy products; no refined or processed foods; no sugar, white flour, coffee, tobacco or alcohol.

Breakfast: 1/2 tsp. Elderberry Extract, 1/2 tsp. Hawthorn Berry tincture, Vitamin E 400 IU, one to two Vitamin B-Complex, B-15 50 mg., Vitamin A 10,000 IU, Lecithin 1200 mg., one capsule Cayenne in middle of meals, Calcium/Magnesium 200/100 mg., Vitamin C 500 mg, two Cleansing formula, two Tibet 28 .

Morning Snack: Vitamin C 500 mg.

Lunch: 1/2 tsp. Hawthorn Berry tincture, Vitamin E 400 IU, one capsule Cayenne in middle of meals, Vitamin C 500 mg., two Tibet 28 .

Mid afternoon snack: Vitamin C 500 mg.

Supper: Same as breakfast.

Note: Vitamin E should start at 100 IU. daily if it has not been used recently, gradually building up to recommended dosage. Make sure bowels are clean.

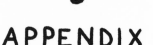

APPENDIX

APPENDICITIS

This condition occurs when the appendix, a short finger-like projection about three inches long attached to the cecum (lower end of the ascending colon), becomes inflamed. Natural Practitioners feel the function of the appendix is to aid in lubrication of the ascending colon. The fecal matter can therefore make the upward trip more easily after entering from the small intestine. The inflammation generally results from some obstruction which is usually caused by constipation or faulty digestion. Pain, generally beginning near the navel, will soon spread to the lower right abdomen and be accompanied by loss of appetite, fever and possibly vomiting or diarrhea. Untreated inflammation may result in a ruptured appendix, causing the infection to spread into the abdominal cavity. This is often fatal.

Recommended Action

First, the colon should be thoroughly cleansed with an enema, repeated periodically as necessary. Take no solid food, drink plenty of liquid and take orally the same herbs as listed below for the enema. They work best in the form of a tea, mixed with fruit juices, or an alkaline (vegetable) broth. Olive oil is beneficial, either added to the enema and/or taken orally to assist in lubricating the colon and removing the obstruction. Demulcent herbs (specifically those for glands) can be made into a healing poultice or fomentation to apply to the affected area repeatedly. It is very important in appendicitis to refrain from using any laxative as this may make the situation even more serious. This is especially true in the case of children, as their tissue is more delicate and more easily ruptured. Captain Roberts suggests one teaspoon of Fluid Extract of Wild Yam in a wineglass of water, one teaspoon Tincture Echinacea in a wineglass of water, and a teaspoon of olive oil taken alternately. He also suggests olive oil rubbed freely into the lower right abdomen.

Single Herbs: Chickweed, Elder flowers, Mullein (hot poultice with Lobelia and Ginger), Lady Slipper root powder (1 teaspoon with 1/2 teaspoon Lobelia herb powder - steep for a few minutes in one cup of water); Echinacea (homeopathic), Ginseng (homeopathic), coffee enemas can be useful also.

ARTERIOSCLEROSIS

This condition involves the buildup of calcium deposits (calcification) on the inside of the artery walls, causing thickening and hardening (sclerosis) of the artery. If the deposits are fatty substances (atheromas), the condition is properly referred to as atherosclerosis. However, both conditions have about the same effect on circulation. High blood pressure (hypertension) is commonly associated with Arteriosclerosis and can cause this condition or, conversely, this condition can cause high blood pressure. The deposits, whether calcium or fatty substances, tend to form in the areas of the arteries that have been weakened by high blood pressure or strain. Narrowing of the arteries forces already high blood pressure even higher. As the arteries become less pliable and less penetrable, ischemia (cell starvation) results due to insufficient circulation to the cells. There is a danger of heart attack, apoplexy or stroke, especially in older people. These are caused when one of the coronary arteries becomes completely obstructed by accumulated deposits or by a blood clot either formed or snagged on the deposit.

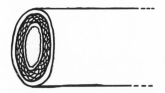

NORMAL ARTERY

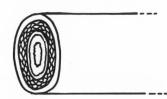

ARTERIOSCLEROSIS

Recommended Action

To strengthen the heart and clean out the artery walls, implement an exercise program, starting slowly and gradually increasing to aerobic activity. The diet should be changed to eliminate all refined starches, white flour, sugar and saturated fats. Reducing the intake of saturated animal fats and animal proteins will help prevent atheromas, which contains high amounts of lipids (fat-related products such as cholesterol and triglycerides). Salt should also be eliminated, and Lecithin, Vitamin C and B Complex should be added to the diet as they will assist in reducing lipid levels in the blood and in strengthening blood vessels.

Single Herbs: Cayenne, Garlic, Siberian Ginseng (antiatherosclerotics and circulatory tonics); Dandelion, Black Radish.

Combinations: Cleansing formula (two - twice daily), Green life (four - three times daily), Tibet 28 (two - twice daily)

Synergistic Vitamins and Minerals: Vitamin B Complex with extra Niacin, B-6, Inositol and Choline, Vitamin C, Vitamin E, Calcium, Magnesium, Chromium and Lecithin.

ARTHRITIS

Arthritis is basically an inflammation of the joints and presents itself in a variety of ways, the two most common being rheumatoid arthritis and osteoarthritis. The former attacks the synovial membranes surrounding the lubricating fluid in the joints and creates stiffness, swelling and often crippling pain. The latter, known as degenerative joint disease, is related to the wear and tear of aging and involves deterioration of the cartilage ends of the bones. This second type usually involves much less pain and little or no swelling. Gout, which occurs more often in overweight people and those who indulge regularly in rich foods and alcohol, is another form of arthritis. It usually occurs in the smaller joints of the feet and hands, generally affecting the big toe. Deposits of crystallized uric acid salt in the joint cause swelling, redness, and a sensation of heat and extreme pain.

Recommended Action

Drink steam-distilled water daily and take a generous portion of herbs capable of dissolving organic deposits of calcium and mineral salts responsible for the symptoms of arthritis. Anchovies, sardines, beef and internal organs of animals (such as kidneys and liver) are all rich in purine (a substance involved in the production of uric acid) and should therefore be avoided by anyone with gouty arthritis. Follow a good natural diet and use periodic juice fasting or cleansing diets to help this condition improve.

Single Herbs: Ma Hueng herb, Chaparral, Devil's Claw, Hydrangea, Irish Moss, Yucca (for dissolving inorganic deposits); Alfalfa, Dandelion root, Comfrey, Licorice root, Bee Pollen (organic nutrients); Saffron (for dissolving uric salts in Gout); Aloe Vera gel or juice, Red Clover, Dulse.

Combinations: Arthritis formula; Bone, Flesh and Cartilage (for dissolving inorganic deposits); Nerve formula (pain relief); Cleansing formula, Lower Bowel Tonic (cleanser and eliminator).

Synergistic Vitamins and Minerals: Vitamin A, B Complex with B-12, B-6, Niacin, Pantothenic acid, Vitamin C, Vitamin E, Calcium, Magnesium, Trace Minerals, Cod or Halibut Liver Oil.

Suggested Program:

Follow Arthritis diet (see Appendix).

One hour before breakfast take one tablespoon of Cod or Halibut Liver oil. This can be mixed with a 2 tablespoons of orange juice or milk. Nothing else, including water, should be taken for half an hour.

Breakfast: Take one tablespoon of apple cider vinegar with one teaspoon of honey in one-third to one cup of warm water at the beginning of breakfast. Take: two Arthritis formula, two B-Complex Vitamin C 500 mg., two Calcium/Magnesium 300/150 mg., one Multi-trace Mineral., 1200 mg. Lecithin.

Morning Snack: Vitamin C 500 mg.

Lunch: Vitamin C 500 mg., one Tbsp. Aloe Vera Gel, one Irish Moss capsule, Vitamin E 100 IU.

Afternoon Snack: Vitamin C 500 mg., two Bee Pollen.

Supper: Same as breakfast.

Evening: Cod or halibut liver oil, as taken before breakfast.

Note: Make sure bowels are clean; if they are not, take Lower Bowel Tonic.

ASTHMA

Asthma is a type of allergic reaction which attacks the respiratory system and is characterized by labored breathing, coughing, wheezing and often a feeling of suffocation. The allergens which can cause asthma generally include such things as dust, pollen, animal hairs, foods and various chemical substances found in both processed foods and air. However, asthmatic attacks may also be set off by emotional stress, as this lessens the body's resistance and increases its sensitivity to allergens in the environment. During an asthma attack, a muscle spasm causes the bands of involuntary muscles, which surround the bronchials (small air passages in the lungs), to constrict. Consequently, the flow of air to the alveoli (tiny air sacs within the lungs) is also restricted. This is often accompanied by the simultaneous swelling of the lining of the air passages, with excessive secretion of mucus into these passages. All these combine to cause even more difficulty. In an effort to expel mucus from the air passages, the body initiates asthmatic coughing, while the wheezing sound comes from air travelling over pockets of mucus in the passages causing them to resonate. Chronic wheezing, not accompanied by asthmatic attacks, could indicate a dietary problem involving excessive amounts of mucus-forming foods and is often accompanied by a mild nervous condition. There is also clinical evidence linking asthma to hypoglycemia.

Recommended Action

For acute attacks take a cup of Elder flower or berry tea; follow this by a 1/4 tsp. of Lobelia Extract and/or Ma Hueng tea or extract as it is also beneficial in relaxing the bronchial muscles. In order to obtain long-term relief it is necessary to remove all mucus-forming foods from the diet. The following supplements are also extremely beneficial:

1. Vitamin A for healthy lungs.
2. B-Complex to strengthen the nervous system.
3. Vitamin C to combat stress factors.
4. Calcium to relax and rebuild the nerves.
5. Potassium to inhibit mucus production.

It is also helpful to use relaxant herbs to prevent constriction of the bronchial muscles, and expectorant herbs to help release and expel mucus. Ephedrine is often used in medical treatment as a bronchiodilator (opens up air passages),

Asthma Case Study

In the case of bronchial , asthmatic and many other lung problems we have found Ma Huang to be an excellent herb; but it is best regulated as in the lung formula. Mrs.V. from Prince Albert, Sask., had such bad asthma that she couldn't sleep properly at nights: "I felt as if I was drowning". But following the outlined program, within a week she could sleep at night and in one and a half months she was breathing normally again. After ten months of following the program she was symptom free, without the supplement, as long as she didn't eat mucus-forming foods.

as is adrenalin. Cortisone is also used in conventional therapy to stimulate adrenal activity. Some natural herbal substitutes for these remedies would be Ma Hueng (in which ephedrine occurs naturally) and Licorice root (which stimulates the adrenals). It is also beneficial to keep the living area and especially the sleeping area quite humid. A vaporizer or humidifier is good and will act as a mild bronchiodilator if you put a few drops of eucalyptus oil in it.

Single Herbs: Ma Hueng (bronchiodilator); Licorice root (expectorant and adrenal stimulant); Slippery Elm, Comfrey, Mullein (demulcents, expectorants, specifics for lungs); Elderberry Extract (potassium, anti-mucus); Lobelia Extract (relaxant, emetic and expectorant); Bee Pollen (see Allergies); Garlic (expectorant).

Combinations: Lung Formula.

Synergistic Vitamins and Minerals: Vitamins A, B- Complex, C, D, E, Calcium, Magnesium, Manganese.

Suggested Program:

Start the program with a 7 - 10 day Inner Cleanse Diet, while avoiding all mucus-forming foods. Diet should emphasize garlic, green vegetables and fresh fruits. Manganese-rich foods are also advisable, some of which are peas, beans, blueberries, nuts and buckwheat. Alternating hot and cold showers have been found quite successful. Take a 3-5 minute hot shower, switching immediately to a cold shower (as cold as possible) for 10-15 seconds. Repeat three times, always ending with a cold shower. Of course plenty of aerobic exercise in clean, non-smoggy air is beneficial.

Supplements:

Breakfast: Two Lung formula, Vitamin A 40,000 IU, Vitamin B-Complex (25-50 mg.) with B-6 25 mg., Pantothenic Acid 50 mg., Vitamin C 500 mg., Vitamin D 1200 IU, Calcium/Magnesium 200/100 mg., Vitamin E 400 IU., two Garlic capsules, Manganese 5 mg. (twice a week for 10 weeks).

Morning Snack: Vitamin C 500 mg.

Lunch: Lung formula, Vitamin C 500 mg., Calcium/ Magnesium 200/100 mg., Vitamin A 20,000 IU.

Afternoon Snack: Vitamin C 500 mg.

Supper: Same as breakfast.

BEDWETTING

Unconscious wetting during sleep by a person over the age of three is clinically termed enuresis, while involuntary urination by a child or adult during waking hours is referred to as incontinence. Infection or inflammation of the urinary tract, worms or other irritants, general weakness and debility, extreme tiredness, drinking too much liquid, eating spicy food which irritates the urinary tract and emotional stress can all cause this problem.

Recommended Action

Refined foods should be eliminated from the diet as they weaken the system. Eat the evening meal no later than 4 or 5 o'clock and do not eat again before bedtime. Especially do not allow liquid the last few hours before bedtime. If thirsty, give fresh fruit, but only if absolutely necessary. Immediately upon arising give plenty of liquids so as to dilute the strength of retained urine. Many cases of enuresis are of an emotional nature. If the parents are confronted in the child's presence with the statement that the child is merely doing it for attention, they will usually state that their child gets all the attention that he needs. At some subconscious level the child realizes that he does indeed get attention, and the enuresis will often cease shortly thereafter.

Single Herbs: Uva-Ursi, Juniper berries, Buchu, Parsley leaves.

Combinations: Kidney Formula.

Synergistic Vitamins and Mineral: Vitamin A (10,000 IU, twice daily), Vitamin B-complex, Vitamin C (500 mg. three times daily), multi-vitamin and minerals.

BLADDER INFECTION

See Kidney and Bladder.

BLEEDING

Bleeding usually refers to the external loss of blood from a blood vessel, while hemorrhage usually refers to the rupture of an internal blood vessel. External bleeding can involve a wide range of severity and include such things as abrasions (scrapes), lacerations (tears), punctures (such as stabbing) or gunshot wounds. In less severe wounds, involving broken or severed capillaries, the blood will flow momentarily in order to wash out the wound, and within a few minutes a clot will begin to form. In more severe wounds, involving a severed vein or artery, the flow of blood will be stronger and more profuse.

Arterial blood is bright red because it contains a high amount of oxygen and is being pumped directly from the heart; it will flow in spurts. On the other hand, venous blood is darker because it is returning from the cells, carrying carbon dioxide rather than oxygen and not being pumped directly; it will flow more steadily. A bruise is an area of mild internal tissue damage where blood released from capillaries has accumulated. The change in color of a bruise from red or purple to brown, green or even yellow before completely disappearing directly results from the hemoglobin in the red blood cells breaking down as the blood elements rebuild the injured tissue.

Recommended Action

The best emergency measure for any bleeding, either internal or external, is a teaspoon of cayenne in a glass of warm water. If bleeding is internal, use a homeostatic herb that is a specific for the particular organ involved. Simmer it in one pint of milk, then drink it slowly. Cayenne, to control the bleeding. Golden Seal, to prevent infection, may be applied directly to minor external wounds. Plantain, comfrey or yarrow (either fresh or powdered) are more beneficial for severe wounds (internal or external). In a case of arterial or venous bleeding, apply direct pressure around the wound and get immediate attention. Generally, bruises are not serious, however, if bruising occurs easily, it signifies fragile, or easily ruptured, blood vessels. This condition can be remedied with a good calcium supplement, and it is advisable to beware of Vitamin C deficiency. Large amounts of bioflavonoids are also usually needed.

Single Herbs: Cayenne, Plantain, Comfrey, Yarrow (vulneraries); Golden Seal root (uterine hemeostatic); Mullein (bowel and lungs); Marshmallow (bladder); Golden Seal, White Oak bark (nose); Gumweed ointment (prevents scarring).

Synergistic Vitamins and Minerals: Vitamin A 20,000 IU., Vitamin C 1000 - 3000 mg., Vitamin E oil over scab area after healing has advanced, Bioflavonoids (250 mg. four - six times daily), Calcium/Magnesium 200/100 mg. daily, Trace Minerals.

BLOOD PRESSURE

See High or Low Blood Pressure.

BOWEL & COLON

Proper functioning of the bowel and colon is essential to good health. The term "bowel" refers to both the large and small intestines, while "colon" refers only to the lower bowel or large intestine. The primary function of the colon is to absorb water and electrolytes and solidify the fecal matter prior to elimination from the body. The bulk of the nutrients is absorbed by the small intestine, with only a small amount of nutrients being absorbed in the ascending and transverse sections of the colon. Fecal deposits adhere to the walls of the intestine and solidify. They are a direct result of a rich diet and refined foods producing varying degrees of chronic constipation. Normal bowel movements become difficult to impossible as the hardened deposits interfere with absorption and immobilize peristaltic muscles.

Recommended Action

Drink copious amounts of steam-distilled or reverse osmosis water and be sure to include plenty of fresh fruits, vegetables, whole grains, nuts and seeds in the diet. Supplementing with additional vegetable fiber may be necessary in some cases. Alfalfa sprouts or tablets are excellent. Lower Bowel Tonic is a good remedy to help rebuild immobilized peristaltic muscles. Highly refined starches and sugars should be eliminated entirely from the diet, while it is advisable to greatly reduce the intake of rich foods and mucus forming foods, such as meat, eggs and dairy products. One of the most common herbs to use for colon problems is Senna, however, long term use of it can become habit forming.

Single Herbs: Alfalfa, Cascara sagrada, Turkey Rhubarb.

Combinations: Lower Bowel Tonic (two tablets three times daily); occasionally Senna and Ginger (3:1 ratio); Psyllax (acts as a bulking poultice for the intestinal tract); Green Life (intestinal detoxifier and oxygenator).

BRONCHITIS

Bronchitis is any inflammation occurring in the mucous membrane which lines the bronchial tubes of the lungs. Coughing, wheezing, spitting up of mucus and difficulty breathing are all the usual symptoms. Acute bronchitis generally results as a complication of infection elsewhere in the respiratory tract, while chronic bronchitis results from protracted lung irritation (i.e., heavy smoking, air pollution or stubborn infection in the throat or lungs). Serious diseases such as emphysema, tuberculosis and lung cancer are usually preceded by bronchitis.

Recommended Action

Hot vapor or steam baths (especially with a little eucalyptus oil) facilitate dilation (opening) of the bronchial passages. Herbs of a demulcent and expectorant nature can be taken orally or applied as hot fomentations to the chest and thoracic area of the spine to obtain relief. If the condition is severe, it

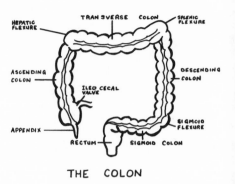

THE COLON

Constipation

Mrs. T. came into my clinic in 1977 with a constipation problem. I suggested Lower Bowel Tonic at a dosage of two capsules, three times daily. This normal dosage wasn't enough so we increased the dosage until she had one full bowel movement daily. Her dosage was an extraordinary four capsules, five times daily. Her biggest question was: ". . . won't I become dependent on these as I have on laxatives and enemas?". I assured her that this wasn't the case with the Lower Bowel Tonic. After one year she only needed twelve to have two movements daily; by two years it was down to six capsules, and by two years seven months she didn't need any to maintain one to two movements daily. Four years later, she only took the Lower Bowel Tonic if she had eaten a very big dinner or if she had eaten improperly for a while (she generally used about three - five a month).

may be necessary to use an emetic which will bring up the excess mucus and relax the throat, stomach and bronchial passages. It is also important to cleanse the bowel and eliminate mucus-forming foods from the diet.

Single Herbs: Ma Hueng, Coltsfoot herb, Mullein, Comfrey, Lobelia, Marshmallow root.

Combinations: Lung formula.

Synergistic Vitamins: Vitamins A, B-Complex, C, D, E, Bioflavonoids, Iron, Manganese, Multi-Vitamins and Minerals.

Suggested Program:

Breakfast: Two Lung formula, Carotene Vitamin A 20,000 - 40,000 IU, Vitamin C 500 mg., Vitamin D 400 IU, Vitamin E 200 IU, Bioflavonoids 200 mg.

Morning Snack: Vitamin C 500 mg., Elderberry Extract 1/2 tsp., Lobelia extract five drops.

Lunch: Two Lung formula, Vitamin C 500 mg.

Afternoon Snack: Same as morning snack.

Supper: Same as breakfast.

BURNS

Burns are the result of exposure to extreme or prolonged heat causing different degrees of damage to the skin. Only the outer layer of skin is affected in first degree burns, which involve redness and discomfort but no actual blistering or destruction of flesh. The next layer of skin may be penetrated by second degree burns, which involve raised blisters, sometimes destroyed hair follicles and sweat glands and often serious infectious complications. Complete destruction of the skin tissue occurs in third degree burns, which involve damage to deeper tissues, leaving the skin either charred or whitened. Sunburns are usually only first degree but may sometimes be second degree burns. Although not severe, they cause great discomfort due to the large surface area they occupy. For serious burns or those covering a large area, medical aid should be sought immediately.

Recommended Action

Regardless of the degree of burn or scald, the best first aid to use is cold water to take the heat out. It is also important to guard against the complications

Aloe works

I was out at my cabin one fall cutting firewood for the winter. I had been chainsawing for about five hours, my arms were quite sore and the chainsaw was very hot. In one of those great moments of complete clumsiness I leaned my hand down onto the exhaust of the saw. My hand started to cook immediately. Before I knew what had happened my right hand had a very severe burn. I immediately soaked my hand in cold water, which, of course, brought the temperature down and gave some quick but very short-lived relief. I then started to prepare an Aloe Vera bath. To do this I put enough Aloe to completely cover my hand into a stainless steel bowl. This bowl I placed into another much larger bowl which was filled with ice. Instant pain relief, but as soon as I took my hand out of the Aloe -instant pain. After several hours of keeping my hand immersed in the Aloe and pain free (with much pain if I dared lift it out again), I began to try to figure out how to sleep leaving my hand in the Aloe. I finally bandaged my hand up in Aloe drenched gauze. My burn healed in what I considered record time with no lack of movement or scarring.

of dehydration, shock and infection. For minor burns, after soaking the burn in cold water to return body temperature to normal, apply a healing salve. (Do not use an oil base salve on open wounds.) Leave it on, only adding to it as necessary until the burn is entirely healed. Use straight Aloe Vera gel or alternate with a salve made of honey, wheat germ oil and olive oil, all of which make good burn salves. Honey salve, with equal parts of honey and wheat germ oil blended with powdered Comfrey, is a very good remedy, but probably the best remedy is pure Aloe Vera gel or juice. Pain can be relieved by bathing with diluted apple cider vinegar, while Vitamin E oil is extremely beneficial to aid the rebuilding of burned tissue (don't put on burn until it has returned to body temperature). To prevent scarring once healing is under way, apply Gumweed ointment or Calendula ointment.

PABA, a B vitamin, taken internally or applied locally, will effectively prevent sunburn. Do not use Vitamin E on burns that are infected or when there is risk of infection, as it can interfere with the infection-fighting ability of the white blood cells.

Single Herbs: Aloe Vera gel, Comfrey ointment, Gumweed ointment.

Synergistic Vitamins and Minerals: Vitamin A 10,000-20,000 IU, B-Complex, PABA 50-100 mg., Vitamin C 3000-5000 mg., Vitamin E 800 IU plus topical application, Zinc 10 mg.

BURSITIS

The synovial bursa are small fluid-filled sacs whose function is to prevent friction between the parts of a joint. Bursitis is the inflammation of this sac. Injury or infection is generally responsible for acute bursitis while chronic bursitis may or may not have obvious causes. Some calcium deposits are inevitably revealed in the troublesome joint when x-rays are taken. Congestion in the transverse colon seems to be associated with bursitis in the neck and shoulder.

Recommended Action

Short-term relief of symptomatic pain can be achieved through the use of fomentations and liniments (Arnica and Cayenne Tinctures). However, a thorough cleansing program and a diet low in mucus are necessary to correct the problem.

Single Herbs: Devil's Claw, Yucca, Cayenne, Arnica tincture.

Combinations: Arthritis formula, Rheumatic formula, Nerve tablets, Lower Bowel Tonic (if constipation associated).

Synergistic Vitamins and Minerals: Vitamin A, B Complex with B-12 and B-6, Niacin, Pantothenic Acid, Vitamin C, Vitamin D, Vitamin E, Calcium, Magnesium, Trace Minerals, Cod or Halibut Liver Oil, Lecithin.

Suggested Program:

Follow program for Arthritis with Arthritis Diet. Add to the program one capsule of Cayenne in the middle of breakfast and supper.

COLITIS

Colitis is an inflammation of the colon (large intestine). It may be simply a mucus condition or it may be ulcerative, with blood as well as mucus showing up in the stool. Diarrhea is common, sometimes alternating with constipation. Loss of weight, anemia, and even toxemia are common complications. Others include hemorrhoids, abscesses, and prolapsis of the colon. Depression and other emotional conditions can precipitate attacks of colitis.

Recommended Action

Limit the diet to juices or pureed fruits and vegetables. Lots of steam-distilled or reverse osmosis water is beneficial, along with the following:

Combinations: Psyllax (soothe colon, aid in ulceration, slow down diarrhea); Lower Bowel Tonic (to tone and strengthen colon); Cleansing formula.

Synergistic Vitamins and Minerals: Vitamin A (20,000 to 40,000 IU); B Complex; Calcium/Magnesium (2 twice daily); Vitamin C (500 mg. twice daily).

Suggested Program:

Start with one tablespoon of Musilax in one cup of tomato juice twice daily (if tomato juice irritates, use other liquid). After three days take one Lower Bowel Tonic daily, increase to one tablet two times daily after one week. In third week add one Cleansing formula. In fourth week add two more Lower Bowel Tonic and one Cleansing. By the fourth week you should be taking: 2 Lower Bowel Tonic twice daily, 1 Cleansing Formula twice daily and you may stop taking Musilax.

CONSTIPATION

See Bowel and Colon.

COUGHS

Coughing is an attempt by the body to dislodge and expel some irritating or obstructing matter from the chest or throat and consists of reflex action of the respiratory muscles accompanied by a blast of air. Demulcent and expectorant herbs help to loosen and break up the offending substance (if it is mucus), so it can then be expelled. Even the most bothersome cough can be helped by drinking a little warm water mixed with one tablespoon of lemon juice and one tablespoon of honey. Antispasmodic herbs are necessary to treat spasmodic coughs since this kind involves irritation of a nerve which then activates the coughing reflex.

Single Herbs: Ma Hueng, Licorice root, Slippery Elm (lozenges), Marshmallow, Mullein, Comfrey (demulcents and expectorants); Lobelia Extract (antispasmodic and expectorant).

Combinations: Lung formula.

Synergistic Vitamins and Minerals: Vitamin A 20,000 - 50,000 IU., Vitamin-B Complex 25-50 mg. ratio, Vitamin C 3000 - 5000 mg., Calcium 20 mg..

When and when not to suppress a cough

Some coughs should be suppressed and some shouldn't. If a cough is full of mucus, we want to encourage the expectoration of the mucus. But if the cough is a dry cough, there is usually some sort of irritation in the throat. With a dry cough try to soothe the throat and thereby stop the cough. Also consider if a throat problem might be caused by drainage from the sinuses.

CRAMPS

Cramps may indicate a mineral imbalance and particularly a deficiency of calcium or magnesium. They consist of spasmodic, involuntary muscle contractions which are generally accompanied by great pain.

Single Herbs: Alfalfa, Cayenne or Cayenne Extract (leg and muscle cramps); Ginger (uterine); Chamomile, Peppermint (stomach); Lobelia Extract, Cramp Bark (antispasmodic).

Combinations: Herbal Calcium (leg and muscle cramps); Female formula (Uterine cramps); Stomach formula (stomach), Lower Bowel Tonic (intestinal).

Synergistic Vitamins and Minerals: Vitamin D 400 IU, B-6 50-100 mg., Pantothenic Acid 100 mg., Calcium Lactate 600-1500 mg., Magnesium Oxide 300-800 mg., Vitamin E 400-1000 IU, Magnesium Phosphate 6-12X tissue salt (four when needed), Multiminerals and trace minerals.

Suggested Program:

If the cramps are intestinal or uterine take a few capsules of Ginger, or a tea of equal parts of Ginger, Blessed Thistle and Cramp Bark. If the cramps are in a large muscle take plenty of Calcium, Magnesium and Magnesium Phosphate tissue salts, and some Tincture of Cayenne for circulation. Rub Cayenne and Arnica Tincture into the area to help ease cramps and to stimulate circulation. B and B tincture, taken orally or mixed into a liniment, is beneficial.

CYSTS

Cysts usually appear just under the surface of the skin and are abnormal sac-like growths which contain fluid or semi-fluid substance. They are also common on the mucous membranes of the body, particularly those of the female reproductive organs. They are distinguishable from tumors, which consist of solid matter, in that they contain mucus, dead tissue debris, pus or even hair, but they are rarely malignant.

Recommended Action

While you are trying to eliminate cysts, the Cleansing Diet should be followed for ten days, alternating with the Daily Diet Regime. It is often beneficial to add in a third cycle of a three-day cleansing fast. Then repeat the cycle. Whole grains are also very beneficial to rid the body of cysts.

Single Herbs: Black Walnut leaves, hulls, bark, or Extract; Burdock, Chaparral.

Combinations: Female formula (cysts in female areas); Green Life, Tibet 28 (cysts anywhere).

Breast Cysts

Mrs. L. came in with three fair size cysts in her left breast. It was suggested that she take two Cleansing formula three times daily; two Female formula three times daily; 400 IU Vitamin E twice daily; a low mucus diet with lots of freshly cooked whole grains. After a month the cysts had reduced in size substantially; after two months they were completely gone.

DIABETES

See Pancreas.

DIAPER RASH

Diaper rash, otherwise known as diaper dermatitis, is a localized skin irritation. It is caused by extensive skin contact with a wet or soiled diaper and can range in severity from mild redness to blistering. It is commonly followed by secondary yeast or bacterial infections.

Recommended Action

Changing the diapers more frequently will avoid further irritation. The skin should be kept clean and dry with air circulating to it as much as possible. Avoid the use of plastic pants. Chickweed or Mullein ointment should be applied to give relief.

Single Herbs: Mullein (topically applied); Oil of Garlic (topically applied);

A Mullein Diaper

Dr. J. R. Christopher tells a story of a very poor woman who couldn't afford proper diapers for her child, and diaper rash was the result. Things got financially worse for the lady so she tried to make diapers out of some big mullein leaves, and to her astonishment the child's diaper rash went away. Both mullein and chickweed ointments are excellent for diaper rash.

Black Walnut Extract (topically applied, especially for yeast infections); Chickweed ointment (emollient); Chamomile tea (wash).

DIARRHEA

Frequent and abnormal liquid bowel movements are indications of this condition. Other body disorders such as colitis, amoebic dysentery, food or chemical poisoning and emotional stress can cause diarrhea. It can also be brought on by infection (either in the digestive tract or elsewhere in the body) or by digestive problems resulting from chemical, hormonal or enzyme deficiencies, or it may occur by itself. If the diet has just been changed to one high in roughage, or fiber, and fresh fruits, diarrhea will often result until the body adjusts. Dehydration, loss of minerals, and loss of water soluble vitamins and beneficial intestinal flora (bacteria) will occur if the condition is not remedied.

Recommended Action

Diarrhea should be treated as a symptom and efforts should be made to determine the cause. It is advisable to replace lost fluid by drinking large quantities of juice or some other liquid. Astringent herbs can be employed both orally and in the form of an enema. If the diarrhea is a result of amoebic dysentery, colitis, emotional stress, food poisoning or any other disorder, it is important to deal with that particular condition specifically. In cases of extreme constipation nothing but water can get through and this condition manifests itself as diarrhea. The obstruction can be removed by the use of an enema, and the peristaltic muscles can be stimulated and gradually rebuilt by the use of appropriate herbs. If there is excessive bleeding of the bowel, make a tea from one ounce mullein leaves simmered in one pint of milk. Strain and drink it immediately after the bowels move. This is an effective remedy and will often achieve results where all else fails. The mullein acts as a homeostatic and demulcent and is held against the membrane walls by the milk which coats them. Make a fresh batch each time and drink the whole thing immediately after each bowel movement until the bleeding stops. In infantile diarrhea the loss of potassium can be serious or even fatal. Mashed banana will supply a large amount of potassium and halt the diarrhea.

Single Herbs: White Oak bark, Red Raspberry (astringent enema); Slippery Elm (astringent and demulcent); Mullein (for bleeding bowel); Fluid Extract of Wild Strawberry, Uva-Ursi (astringent).

Combinations: "Po Chai", Psyllax.

DIGESTION

Digestion is a process of breaking down the foods we eat and changing them into a form which is easily assimilated by the body's cells to use for energy, tissue replacement and growth. The digestive process begins in the mouth. All food should be thoroughly chewed to break fibers and other hard matter apart. Chewing is also important to ensure that the first of the digestive enzymes found in the saliva are properly mixed in with the food. The next stage of digestion takes place in the stomach, where more enzymes are added along with HCl. Only alcohol, water, some vitamin C and certain sugars are absorbed in the stomach. The food moves on to the small intestine where additional enzymes are secreted, from both the pancreas and the small intestine itself. Here, bile which comes from the liver, is also added and acts as an alkalizer and laxative and assists in the breakdown of fats. Most of the absorption of nutrients takes place in the small intestine; the nutrients are then carried by the blood to the cells. The waste products of digestion are passed along to the large intestine, where some minerals and water are reabsorbed and finally the waste is excreted. In this long chain of events, we often see many symptomatic problems manifested. These can include heartburn, gas, acid indigestion, constipation, diarrhea, vomiting, colic and other conditions (treated individually under the particular heading for that problem). The digestive system must be functioning properly if we are to get the healthy nutrients we need into our bodies. Otherwise it is possible to starve in the midst of plenty while the much-needed vitamins and herbs are flushed away.

Poor Digestion

Probably 80% of the people that come into my clinic have some sort of digestive problem. The most common is the lack of proper enzymes and gastric juice production. This is often caused by simply eating too fast for many years, resulting first in low hydrochloric acid production in the stomach. Giving the person Stomach Formula will usually build up the stomach in three to nine months, at which time we can stop its usage. In more stubborn cases we often have to give the person some digestive enzymes during the meal for the first while to "prime the pump", as it were.

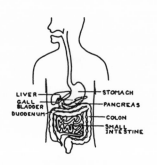

Recommended Action

Overeating, eating in a rushed or excited state, improper mastication (chewing) and salivation, and poor food combinations (eating the wrong foods together) are the most common causes of digestive problems. The solutions are obviously simple: never overeat, eat moderate amounts and only when hungry, take the time to eat in a relaxed state, avoid eating if you are rushed or emotionally upset, chew each mouthful slowly and thoroughly and avoid "inhaling" food. Finally, foods such as refined starches and sugars contribute to poor digestion and putrefaction, resulting in gas and other improper acid balances in the stomach, and so should be avoided. To help correct the acid balance in the stomach (whether too high or too low) take 1 tablespoon of apple cider vinegar in a glass of warm water sweetened with 1 teaspoon honey, before meals. Fermented foods such as yogurt, miso and sauerkraut can aid digestion and help prevent intestinal putrefaction. Garlic and Bee Pollen are also beneficial in preventing putrefaction and will help eliminate gas. Herbs of a stomachic and aromatic nature will aid digestion, while those that are carminative will eliminate gas, and herbs such as comfrey, which is demulcent in nature, will soothe the mucous membranes of the digestive tract.

Single Herbs: Catnip, Chamomile, Ginger (aromatics); Cayenne, Ginseng, Peppermint (stomachic); Fennel, Fenugreek, Wild Yam (carminative); Saffron, Meadow Sweet (antacid); Papaya Leaves (digestive enzyme), Garlic, Bee Pollen, Comfrey.

Combinations: Stomach formula.

Synergistic Vitamins and Minerals: B-Complex, Digestive enzymes.

Suggested Program:

Although their use can become habit forming, starting off with digestive enzymes specific to the problem, (usually one with the two major daily meals) can add to a herbal program. The enzymes will help to digest the herbs more fully so the rest of the digestive system can gradually take over with its own enzymes, allowing the elimination of those taken orally. This process usually takes about one - two months. Working with the digestion is often the best place to start a general herbal building program. Take one Stomach formula before two meals daily, two Lower Bowel Tonic twice daily from the start of the program.

DIVERTICULITIS

Diverticulitis occurs when diverticula (small pouch-like sacs found in mucous membranes, particularly those of the large intestine) become inflamed. These pouches are abnormal but pose no real health problem by themselves. However, if food particles become entrapped in them, which is a common occurrence, inflammation will result. It is usually accompanied by fever, constipation, severe abdominal pain and occasionally blood in the stool. It is possible for the intestinal passage to become partially blocked in some cases.

Recommended Action

See treatment for Colitis.

Synergistic Vitamins and Minerals: Folic acid (one mg. daily), Multiple minerals and vitamins (two daily), Garlic oil capsules, Whey powder (one tablespoon with each meal), Cod Liver oil (two tablespoons daily).

DIZZINESS

Dizziness is characterized by feelings of giddiness, unsteadiness, lightheadedness or faintness. In some cases it is a normal reaction to a change in atmosphere, such as the reduced amount of oxygen at higher altitudes. It can also indicate constipation, menstrual problems, high or low blood pressure, hypoglycemia, anemia, diabetes, arteriosclerosis or temporary lack of circulation to the brain. Vertigo is the medical term for the sensation of spinning or falling, or of standing still while the surrounding objects seem to be moving. Often it goes hand in hand with nausea, vomiting, perspiration and headache. It invariably originates in the inner ear, the body's equilibrium center (sense of balance). Occasionally brain tumors are responsible for the problem, but more often it is a result of an ear infection or head injury.

Recommended Action

It is first necessary to determine if dizziness is merely a symptom of another problem in order to find and rectify the cause. In a multitude of situations simple constipation is the cause, especially if headaches are also present and relief from the dizzy sensation can be obtained by the use of stimulant herbs. In a true case of vertigo, the cause must again be determined and steps taken to relieve any accompanying nausea and vomiting. Nervine herbs can help to restore function of the inner ear. Every night before retiring put a few drops of garlic oil in each ear; follow this with a few drops of ear and nerve drops (B & B Tincture). A three-day cleansing fast can also be helpful.

Single Herbs: Cayenne, Peppermint, Dandelion root (for relief of dizziness).

Combinations: B & B Tincture, Nerve Formula.

Synergistic Vitamins and Minerals: B complex (50 mg. ratio, two times daily), B6 (150 mg, two times daily), Vitamin C (1,000 mg. daily).

EARACHES AND EAR INFECTIONS

These problems are extremely common especially in young children, who will often indicate the presence of a problem by pulling or rubbing their ears when they are unable to speak. Earaches are often symptoms of a number of other conditions such as head injuries, infection of the eyes, ears, nose, throat or glandular system. Several home remedies are available to relieve the pain. If the pain is caused by infection, the source should be determined. Injury, intrusion of foreign matter, or such things as swimming in contaminated water usually cause outer ear infections (from the eardrum outward). Infections which spread from the nose and throat through the eustachian tubes usually cause middle ear infections (the small cavity on the inside of the eardrum). This type often involves diminished hearing and a feeling of fullness in the ear along with pain and fever. It is inner ear infections which upset the body's equillibrium center causing dizziness, nausea, vomiting and partial or total loss of hearing. This is often the result of a spreading middle ear infection (otitis media) or meningitis.

Recommended Action

Immediate relief from the pain of earache can be obtained by placing ice packs on the affected ear. Always treat both ears when dealing with infection; this will keep the infection from spreading from one ear to the other. To relieve pain and drain out infection, lightly bake an onion cut in half; take the warm onion and place half over each ear and hold in place overnight with a large wrapped bandage, or use a herbal fomentation. Middle and inner ear problems are helped by the insertion of a few drops of garlic oil followed by ear and nerve drops in each ear. Herbs which fight infection should also be taken orally.

Single Herbs: Chamomile, Hops, Mullein (for fomentations over the ears); Oil of Garlic, Lobelia Extract (ear drops); Golden Seal (infection).

Combinations: Three parts Mullein and one part Lobelia used as an external fomentation. B & B Tincture (3 drops) followed by Garlic oil (3 drops) in ear for six nights, on the seventh night rinse ear with equal parts apple cider vinegar and water using an ear syringe.

Synergistic Vitamins and Minerals: Vitamin A (20,000 IU daily); Vitamin C (2,000 mg. daily); Calcium/Magnesium plus D (two twice daily).

EDEMA

Edema (dropsy) is an abnormal accumulation of fluid in the body tissues and it occurs in a variety of forms: Dutaneous dropsy is caused by impaired venous circulation, especially in the extremities. Because the blood is moving slowly, it accumulates and exerts an outward pressure on the walls of the vein. When this pressure becomes greater than the inward osmotic pressure, fluids from the blood escape into the intercellular spaces and cause the characteristic swelling of legs, hands, etc. Pulmonary edema (cardiac dropsy) is caused by failure of the heart to pump blood from the lungs at an adequate rate. This causes pressure in the pulmonary veins, forcing fluid into the lungs. In kidney-related edema, severe loss of blood plasma protein in the urine causes the reverse osmotic pressure and subsequent water retention.

Recommended Action

The solution to all these forms of edema lies in the kidneys and lymphatic system. Most of the excess fluid can be eliminated through the kidneys with the assistance of diuretic herbs and a glandular cleanser. Vapor baths and diaphoretics will also help eliminate a significant portion through the skin. Apply diuretics and diaphoretics as fomentations over affected areas and take them orally also to achieve relief. Avoid salt, meats, pastries, etc. in the diet.

Single Herbs: Parsley, Juniper berries, Gravel root (diuretics).

Combinations: Kidney formula, Parsley/Raspberry leaf tea (1 tsp. of each in 1 cup boiled water); 3 parts Mullein to one part Lobelia (as tea and fomentation).

Synergistic Vitamins and Minerals: B-complex (25 mg.) B6 (50 - 200 mg.); Vitamin C (2,000 - 5,000 mg.), Potassium gluconate, Bromelain (pineapple enzyme).

Suggested Program:

A juice fast is very beneficial for this. The best juices include cucumber, pine-apple and watermelon. (The fast should include only one of the above). Lymphatic drainage massages, done by a professional, are very beneficial as are body bouncers (small trampolines) when used for fifteen minutes daily. Take two Kidney formula three times daily along with parsley and red raspberry leaf tea and Mullein and Lobelia tea daily.

FATIGUE

This is a feeling of mental or physical tiredness which may be the result of physical exertion, mental or emotional stress, rapid weight loss or boredom. On the other hand, it is possible that fatigue is a symptom of anemia, hypoglycemia, nutritional deficiency, obesity or acute infectious disease. Headache, backache, indigestion or general irritability may often accompany fatigue. Cross reference should be made to the above subjects if any of these are suspected.

Recommended Action

The specific underlying disorder must be discovered and dealt with before long term relief can be obtained. A period of rest should follow exercise, perhaps a much needed change will relieve boredom, while detoxification and nutritional supplementation may help in cases of rapid weight loss.

Single Herb: Siberian ginseng, Chinese ginseng, Gotu Kola, Fo-ti-tieng.

Synergistic Vitamins and Minerals: B-complex, Multiple minerals.

FEVERS

Fever can be brought on by a number of causes but is usually related to bacterial or viral infections. Invading micro-organisms and the toxins they release, combined with an excessive accumulation of toxic wastes, upset the body's temperature control mechanism in the hypothalamus (located centrally at the base of the brain), causing abnormally high body temperatures. Natural Healers suggest that these "germs" are rather like little garbage men which feed on and dispose of the accumulated toxic material. Once these wastes are cleaned up, the bacteria begin to die of starvation and are eliminated from the body through discharges and excretions. The fever then breaks and the body enters the recovery stage.

Recommended Action

Usually it is best to encourage and assist a fever, unless it becomes excessively high (about 103 F.). In this case use febrifuges such as Yarrow, Black Walnut, Blessed Thistle, Chamomile, Fenugreek, Lobelia or Thyme. Applying plenty of moist heat is beneficial in fevers. Consider the example of a desert and a jungle: it is apparent that dry heat does not support much life, while moist heat germinates and gives life. Often if the diet is restricted to liquids and the bowels are relieved as soon as a fever is apparent, the fever will break. This in itself can turn into a fairly thorough cleansing. So, a fever can often be a blessing in disguise. It is always advisable to ingest large quantities of liquid. A good tea is Chamomole. If the fever does not subside take the following steps: Use a herbal enema of Catnip, Sage or Red Raspberry tea to help the bowels move if constipation is present. After the bowel is cleaned, use pressed or finely grated garlic in one-half pint of distilled water and one-half pint of apple cider vinegar taken as an injection or an enema. Follow this with a hot bath to which one ounce each of Cayenne, Ginger and dry mustard has been added. This will stimulate the system and promote perspiration. To assist the fever and allay thirst, take warm (never cold) diaphoretic teas such as Yarrow, Catnip, Chamomile, Blessed Thistle or Sage while in the bath. To prevent fainting while in the bath, place a cold towel or washcloth on the forehead. Immediately upon stepping out of the bath, wrap a large double cotton white sheet (soaked in COLD water) around the body and pin it so that only the head and feet can be seen. Next, put the individual in bed, still in the sheet and cover well with wool blankets. Oil the feet well all the way up to the ankles with olive oil then apply a paste of grated garlic and vaseline (half and half) to the soles of the feet only. Use a length of gauze bandage to cover the sole of the foot where the paste is and use a large sock to hold everything in place. Finally pin the bottom of the cold wet sheet closed to form a sack. In the morning the fever will have broken. The sheet will have dried from the heat of the fever and will often be stained by toxic waste that was eliminated with the perspiration.

Single Herbs: Yarrow, Blessed Thistle, Black Walnut, Chamomile, Fenugreek, Raspberry (Diaphoretics).

No Vitamins or Minerals should be taken during fever.

Refer to Daily Food Regime after the fever has broken, for a building program.

FOOD POISONING

Certain bacteria such as staphylococcus, streptococcus, salmonella, shigella and the clostridium bacteria are responsible for food poisoning. The contamination generally is a result of improper food handling and preparation. Using aluminum or unglazed ceramic earthenware for cooking can also cause symptoms like food poisoning and so should be avoided at all costs.

Recommended Action

Use an emetic to empty the stomach of its contaminated contents so that they will not be further assimilated into the system. Ipecac is commonly used, but a large dose (l tsp. - 1 Tbsp.) of Lobelia is unsurpassed for results. Follow this treatment with a quantity of juice and/or distilled water to dilute the toxins that were already absorbed by the system. It is best to follow food poisonings with one day of juice fast, followed by five days of inner cleanse diet (refer to appendix).

Single Herbs: Ipecac, Lobelia (Emetics).

FRACTURES

Injury, rather than disease, is the usual cause of broken bones or fractures.

Recommended Action

Follow the usual first aid procedures: make sure breathing is unobstructed, guard against shock, control bleeding by the application of direct pressure when necessary, and prevent unnecessary movement of the fractured part. Knitting and healing will take place more readily if the following herbal aids are used after the bone has been set.

Single Herbs: Comfrey, Aloe Vera, Oatstraw.

Synergistic Vitamins and Minerals : Vitamin A 20,000 IU, B-Formula (two, twice daily), Vitamin C (500 mg., six times daily), Vitamin D (800 IU, twice daily), Calcium (1000 mg. daily), Magnesium (500 mg., daily), Multiple minerals (two twice daily), trace minerals (two tablets twice daily).

GOUT

See Arthritis.

GRAVEL AND STONES

Gravel and stones are found most often in the gall bladder and in the kidney (renal calculi). Those formed in the gall bladder are chiefly cholestrol, indicating a toxic mucus condition that causes precipitation and hardening of this normally soluble lipid (fatty substance). In both situations the organ and its passages become blocked and the mucous membranes can become torn by the jagged edges of the stones. Infection and considerable pain are the usual results.

Recommended Action

Hydrangea root, Juniper Tincture and Gravel Root are the best solvents for kidney stones. Burdock seed and large amounts of fresh carrot juice are also good. Abstaining from solid food and drinking large quantities of juices and especially Parsley root tea (by the quart) will speed results. (Do not use this treatment if pregnant) In the case of gallstones, fast for two to three days. Take a large glass of prune juice each morning to keep the bowels free and moving. During the day drink plenty of apple juice and reverse osmosis or distilled water. In the evening prepare one cup of olive oil and one cup of fresh squeezed lemon juice; drink six tablespoons of this, thoroughly mixed, every 15 minutes until it is finished, (refer to Liver Flush in Appendix). The stones will then be passed in the stool. It is best to precede this flushing drink with one month of the Liver Formula (two, three times daily). This procedure should be followed with another month of Liver formula. DO NOT DO LIVER FLUSH if liver is in a very acute state.

Single Herbs: Hydrangea root, Gravel root, Uva-Ursi, Parsley root (kidney stone solvents).

Combinations: Kidney Formula, Liver Formula.

Synergistic Vitamins and Minerals: Vitamin A 10,000 IU, Choline 500 mg. (essential for proper fat metabolism), Inositol 500 mg. (involved in cholesterol metabolism), Biotin 25 mcg. (involved in fat assimilation), B-complex (including B-12), C complex, Vitamin E 600 IU, Vitamin D 5,000 IU a week, Lecithin 2,400 mg. twice daily.

HALITOSIS

Halitosis, commonly known as bad breath, is caused by many factors, usually unrelated to the mouth. Although periodontal disease and dental caries can produce odour causing bacteria, regular cleansing of the teeth, gums and tongue can usually overcome this problem. More commonly, halitosis indicates a serious underlying problem involving chemical and metabolic changes within the body. The acetone breath' of diabetic acidosis, the premenstrual halitosis found in many women and the chronic bad breath afflicting millions with gastro-intestinal problems and chronic constipation are all examples of this type of problem. Masking the odour of bad breath with mouthwash is the equivalent of using an air freshener to solve the problem of a backed-up sewer.

Recommended Action

It is most important to avoid constipation, keeping the bowels regular and rebuilding them with the proper herbs. Exercise and a low mucus diet are also helpful. Concentrated alfalfa or liquid chlorophyll taken daily will sweeten the stomach and intestinal tract. Drinking plenty of distilled water daily is often the only solution necessary for some people. Short-term symptomatic relief can be obtained through the use of Cloves, Parsley and Watercress rather than a commercial mouthwash. After a meal heavy in a food such as garlic, we can simply suck on cloves to have sweet-smelling breath.

Single Herbs: Cloves, Parsley, Watercress (breath fresheners); Alfalfa.

Combinations: Lower Bowel Tonic (to stimulate and rebuild the colon), Stomach Formula.

Synergistic Vitamins and Mineral: B-6 50 mg., C- complex 500 mg. twice daily, Zinc 15-30 mg. daily.

HAYFEVER

See Allergies.

HEADACHES

Headaches are most frequently caused by emotional stress or nervous tension but are also symptoms of poor circulation, digestive disturbance, poor ventilation or improper respiration, anemia, hypoglycemia, general infection or head injury. Chronic constipation is one of the most common causes of recurring headaches. Migraine headaches, which are usually accompanied by nausea, vomiting and visual disturbance, result from unusual constriction of the arteries to the brain, leading to a kind of cellular starvation (ischemia). The dilation of the blood vessels causes the typical throbbing pain.

Recommended Action

Realize that headaches only indicate a deeper problem and while anodyne and sedative herbs can help to relax tense nerves and relieve pain, they do not solve the problem. Use the Lower Bowel Tonic to relieve the bowels if constipation is present (enemas should be reserved for emergencies). If the stomach is the source of the problem, use an emetic to empty it. The most effective solution to any headache is rest, and hops, peppermint and chamomile teas will usually induce a restful sleep.

Single Herbs: Lobelia Extract (relaxant, sedative in small amounts, emetic in large amounts); Ginger (for menstrual problems); Hops (sedative, nervine to produce sleep).

Combinations: Nerve tablets (pain), Lower Bowel Tonic (constipation), Muscle Relaxing Formula (general tension).

Synergistic Vitamins and Minerals: B-complex, C-complex, Calcium, Magnesium, Magnesium Phosphate (6x) tissue salt.

HEART

Improper diet and a lack of exercise are common causes of heart problems. The heart becomes overburdened as a result of poor circulation, a bloodstream loaded with impurities and a sluggish system. Our sedentary lifestyles saddle the heart muscle with unnecessary adipose (fatty) tissue, and the extra layers of fat on the body require many more miles of capillaries to supply blood and nutrients to the superfluous cells. The chances of heart failure or of acute heart attack are increased by arteriosclerosis and high blood pressure.

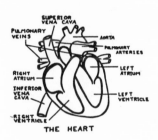

THE HEART

Recommended Action

A teaspoon of Cayenne pepper in a glass of warm water is an effective first aid remedy for an acute heart attack. If the victim is still conscious, breathing and able to drink it, this will regulate the heartbeat. If Cayenne is unavailable, black pepper may be substituted but requires three times as much to achieve the same results. Regular and vigorous exercise is the primary preventative heart care measure. Remember to start off slowly! It is also important to avoid salt, sugar, alcohol, coffee, meat and all refined carbohydrates in the diet. Supplements such as Vitamin E and Lecithin are very beneficial to the heart, and potassium is critical to the proper function of all muscles, including the heart. Daily doses of Elderberry Extract will supply the necessary potassium. Cayenne and Hawthorn berry are the two most important foods for the heart. A malfunctioning thyroid gland is often linked with heart and circulatory problems. In a sense this is the master regulator of all the body's systems and so should be fed and strengthened with appropriate herbs.

Single Herbs: Cayenne, Cayenne Extract, Garlic, Hawthorn Berry, Elderberry Extract.

Synergistic Vitamins and Minerals: Vitamins B-3, B-6, B-Complex, B-15, C, E, Selenium, Calcium/Magnesium, Potassium, Zinc, Copper, Chromium.

Suggested Program:

One of the most important causes of circulatory problems is free radical degeneration of the arterial walls. This degeneration puts a large strain on the heart and all of the following foods have the potential to enhance free radicals and should therefore be avoided:

preservatives, food dyes, partly saturated vegetable oils (especially margarine), rancid oils, chlorinated water, cola drinks, high sugar beverages, coffee, tea (most herb teas are alright), table salt (including sea salt), alcohol, protein-carbohydrate combinations, smoke, cooking with vegetable oils.

The following points should also be adhered to:
1. Roughage should always be present.
2. Meals should be small and fairly frequent. Avoid large meals.
3. Food should be chewed extremely well.

Breakfast - a grain with:
a) one tablespoon of soy lecithin
b) one tablespoon of wheat germ oil (make sure oils aren't rancid)
c) one teaspoon engevita yeast

SUPPLEMENTS: 1 Multi-Mineral
1 Multi Vitamin and Mineral
2 B-Complex
500 mg. C-complex
50 mg. B-15
50 mg. Selenium
1 Calcium/Magnesium tablet
1 tsp. Hawthorn Berry tincture
1 tsp. Cayenne Pepper
1 garlic/parsley tablet
2 Tibet 28

Lunch: a salad or soup.

SUPPLEMENTS: 400 IU Vitamin E (start with 100 IU and build up) 500 mg. C-complex

Supper: a salad with grains, lightly cooked vegetables and/or a little white meat.

SUPPLEMENTS: Same as at breakfast.

Before retiring: 400 IU Vitamin E. (gradually build up to 400 IU)

HEMORRHOIDS

Often known as "piles", this condition involves varicose (enlarged) veins of the anal or rectal area. Weak blood vessels in that area, constipation, straining during elimination, a lifestyle that involves too much sitting and a calcium deficiency are indicated in this situation. They are usually accompanied by itching, and if the condition is uncared for, prolapsus of the anal wall, rupture of small veins and secondary infection may result.

Recommended Action

It is very important to avoid constipation. Change to a diet low in mucus and use the Lower Bowel Tonic. Regular exercise and drinking plenty of steam-distilled or reverse osmosis water daily will help. Apply Vitamin E or wheat germ oil to the area; they may be taken orally as well. Even better results will be found using Plantain ointment and suppositories. A White Oak Bark and Collinsonia root enema has been shown to be useful in this condition.

Single Herbs: Collinsonia Root, Garlic, Mullein, Plantain, White Oak Bark.

Combinations: Lower Bowel Tonic.

Good-bye Hemmorhoids

The best herb for hemmorhoids is Collinsonia root which has the ability to work as an astringent on varicose veins. To avoid hemmorhoids the bowels must be kept active. Pile ointment and suppositories can help avoid the irritation, as can plantain ointment.

HIGH BLOOD PRESSURE

Arteriosclerosis, obesity, stress, excessive salt intake, nervous tension, kidney malfunction and many other factors make it necessary for the heart to work harder in order to pump blood and nutrients to the various body parts. In an attempt to defend itself and correct the situation, the body responds with high blood pressure, otherwise known as hypertension. As this is a symptomatic condition, an attempt to identify and resolve the cause is necessary before attempting to eliminate the symptom.

Recommended Action

Herbs like Cayenne, Garlic, Sassafras and the herbal formula Padma 28 dissolve and remove deposits of precipitated impurities. Avoid mucus forming foods which clog up the bloodstream. It is also wise to avoid overeating, tension and stress, and to eliminate any excess weight. Juice fasts are beneficial if properly conducted. Ensure that the heart and circulatory system are properly nourished. For more information see Heart and Arteriosclerosis.

High Blood Pressure

Over the years there have been many cases of people coming in with high blood pressure. Mr. G. is a good example. He had a blood pressure of 180/120. He took one capsule of cayenne pepper during meals, one garlic/parsley capsule twice daily, one Liver Formula twice daily, 2000 mg. Vitamin C (with 1000 mg. Bioflavinoids), 200IU Vitamin E. His diet excluded all dairy and flour products, salt, fried foods and preservatives. We suggested that he eat lots of whole grains and raw vegetables. In three months his blood pressure was down to 150/100, and in nine months it was 135/90, at which time we slowly lowered his therapy.

Single Herbs: Cayenne or Cayenne Extract, Garlic, Hawthorn Berry Syrup or Tincture, Elderberry Extract.

Synergistic Vitamins and Minerals: Vitamin C (500 mg, two to six times daily); Bioflavonoids (250 mg. two to six times daily); Vitamin E (start with 100 IU gradually increasing to 400 - 800 IU daily); Lecithin (1200 mg. two times daily); Calcium (500 mg.); Magnesium (200 - 500 mg.); Multivitamin and minerals.

HICCUPS

Spasmodic contractions of the diaphragm cause sudden inhalation, followed by a sudden closing of the glottis which produces the "hic" sound. Irritation of the phrenic nerves controlling the diaphragm causes the condition, the irritation often being an overloaded stomach or a sudden emotional change. Singultus is the clinical term for hiccups.

Recommended Action

To relax the nerves and relieve contractions take a few drops of Lobelie Extract on the tongue or in a glass of water.

Single Herbs: Lobelia Extract.

HORMONE IMBALANCE

Hormones and Hair Loss

Hormone imbalances are often responsible for hair loss in both men and women. Women often start to lose hair between eight and fourteen months after delivering a child. This can usually be traced to a hormone imbalance. The loss of hair in men can be a multi-facetted cause, but one fairly common one is an excess of male hormones. In both men and women the reversal of hair loss, if arrested at an early stage, can often be achieved by taking herbal supplements. A good program would be two Female Formula, three times daily; two multi-minerals, twice daily; green lipped mussels, two capsules twice daily; Vitamin E 400 IU daily; plenty of grains, fruits and fresh vegetables.

If one or more of the endocrine glands (pineal, pituitary, thyroid, parathyroid, pancreas, adrenal or reproductive) becomes over- or underactive, hormone imbalances result. Hormones are the chemical regulators of the body's systems and are produced by the aforementioned glands. Major body functions become upset when any one of the above glands produces too much or too little of a particular hormone in relation to others. Often the results can be disastrous.

Recommended Action

Avoid all refined carbohydrates as these have a tendency to throw the glandular machinery off balance. For herbal hormone supplements use those in the following paragraphs.

Single Herbs: Alfalfa (pituitary); Licorice root (adrenals); Cedar Berries (pancreas); Kelp (thyroid); Mullein (all glands); Ginseng, Sarsaparilla (male); Dong Quai, Blessed Thistle, Black Cohosh (female).

Combinations: Female Formula (for males and females, especially during puberty, pregnancy, menopause, male change of life, and after stopping birth control pills).

Synergistic Vitamins and Minerals: Vitamin A, B- Complex, B-6 (75 mg. daily), Zinc, Calcium, Magnesium.

HYPOGLYCEMIA

Hypoglycemia is defined as a low level of glucose (blood sugar) in the bloodstream. It can be caused by an overproduction of insulin or by a malfunction of the adrenal glands. The former results in a too rapid utilization of glucose by the body's cells, while the latter results in overstressed adrenal glands.

A person with low blood sugar will usually show one or more of the following symptoms: a strong craving for sweets or starches; emotional ups and downs; tiredness most of the time, especially in the late afternoon or after eating; stress; easy blow-ups; tiredness upon waking, even with a full night's sleep; difficulty in getting to sleep even when tired; frequent headaches. Hypoglycemia is extremely common in North America because of both our diets and our stress levels. Some authorities estimate it to affect as much as 60% of the population!

Recommended Action

The most important things for low blood sugar (LBS) is to avoid sweets, alleviate the stress, and lessen the overactivity of the pancreas. One of the most common therapies on the market is a high protien diet. I am strongly against this in most cases, and in fact, I feel this type of therapy can often lead to diabetes by overstimulating the system. The therapy that I strongly support is a high proportion of complex carbohydrates. In the Appendix you will find the Complex Carbohydrate Diet that we suggest for people with LBS problems. It is quite important for these people to eat regularly, so we suggest three meals a day with three snacks. Surprisingly; in doing so a person will often lose rather than gain weight.

Single Herbs: Cedar Berries (pancreas); Licorice Root, Uva-Ursi leaves (adrenals).

Combinations: Glucose Formula, Adrenal Stress.

Synergistic Vitamins and Minerals: B-complex, Vitamin C, Vitamin E, Multi-vitamins and minerals, Nucleic acid, Chromium.

Low Blood Sugar

If the accompanying suggested program is followed along with the complex carbohydrate diet in the Appendix and stress levels are lowered, the average hypoglycemic will be able to be symptom free with just a very few maintenance supplements in 12-18 months. If reflexology is added to the program with counselling feedback every two to three weeks the same results can usually be obtained in six to nine months.

Suggested Program:

Follow the Complex Carbohydrate Diet (see Appendix).

Breakfast: 2 Vitamin B-complex
   2 Glucose Formula
   1 Adrenal Stress
   1 Multi-vitamin and mineral
   1 Chromium (if indicated)
   1 Nucleic acid (in quite bad cases)

Morning Snack: 500 mg. Vitamin C

Lunch: 400 IU Vitamin E
   500 mg. Vitamin C
   2 Glucose Formula

Afternoon Snack: 500 mg. Vitamin C

Supper: Same as breakfast

Evening snack: 500 mg. Vitamin C

IMPOTENCE AND FRIGIDITY

Male Impotence

The occurrence of male impotence is much higher than most people think. Here is an example: A fairly successful businessman, in his mid-forties, under too much stress, complains that his sex life isn't what it used to be. In fact, his wife is starting to complain about it. He started taking Ginseng, Vitamin E 400IU twice daily, Kidney formula (two twice daily), and a specially formulated bee pollen called Melbrosia. In his diet he eliminated all preservatives, food dyes, simple carbohydrates and fried foods. Within one month his wife stopped complaining; in two months they were thanking me.

The term impotence is usually used in reference to males and means either the lack of desire or the inability to perform satisfactorily in spite of desire. The term frigidity is usually used in reference to females to indicate the same condition, but may also be used to describe a female totally lacking in interest. The problem for either sex is often psychological in nature and, ironically, is found with increasing frequency in our "liberated" society. It is also possible, however, for it to be due to nutritional and metabolic imbalances or to physical injury.

Recommended Action

If physical injury is not the problem, change to a diet as follows: avoid all refined carbohydrates and eat mainly fresh fruits and vegetables, whole grains, nuts and seeds. Take Vitamin E, wheat germ oil, Ginseng or Siberian Ginseng as a supplement, and drink plenty of distilled or reverse osmosis water.

Single herbs: Ginseng (stimulates all endocrine glands), Bee Pollen (builds up both male and female organs), Orchid (strengthens sexual desires, especially in males), Buchu (strengthens prostate).

Combinations: Female Formula (hormone balancer for both males and females); Adrenal Stress (stimulates sexual activity); Kidney Formula (strengthen male organs); Melbrosia (male or female).

Synergistic Vitamins and Minerals: Vitamin A (10,000 IU twice daily), B-complex, B-6 (50 - 75 mg.), PABA (100 mg.), Vitamin C (500 mg. three times daily), Vitamin E (200 - 600 IU), Zinc (25 75 mg.), Gland concentrates.

INFECTION

Bacteria, viruses or fungi are usually present in the environment and in the body itself. By themselves these micro-organisms pose no serious threat, but when they begin to multiply in accumulated toxic wastes or deteriorating tissue, infection is said to exist. The blood rushes in to supply white blood cells and other elements in an attempt to contain the infection and repair damaged tissue. This results in the characteristic redness and swelling of inflammation.

Recommended Action

Disease germs serve a useful role in cleaning up the internal environment and recycling wastes, but it is most important that they be kept under control. Antiseptic and antibiotic herbs, as well as anthelmintics and febrifuges, are used for this purpose. Refer to specific section for infections in those areas.

Single Herbs: Golden Seal, Echinacea, Myrrh (antiseptic); Garlic (antibiotic); Black Walnut (anthelmintic); Thyme, Fenugreek (febrifuges).

Combinations: Cleansing Formula.

Synergistic Vitamins and Minerals: Vitamin A (20,000 IU twice daily), Vitamin C (500 mg. six times daily).

INSOMNIA

The inability to fall asleep or to stay asleep long enough to obtain sufficient rest is called insomnia, and is often caused by emotional stress, nervous tension, physical aches and pains, meals eaten late at night, mental activity late at night, and stimulants such as are found in coffee, tea, and cola drinks. Hypoglycemia or adrenal exhaustion will often manifested as insomnia.

Recommended Action

Avoid all drugs and sleeping pills, as they not only create an unnatural dependence but also further disturb the dream pattern and can cause neurosis. Avoid late meals and mental activity and make an effort not to worry about the problem as this will only make it worse. Try taking a leisurely walk (especially barefoot, to discharge the static electricity built up in the body during the day), a warm bath or a meditation before bed. These measures can help to remove the insomnia and establish new patterns of restful sleep. Refer also to "Hypoglycemia" for treatment when this apparently is the prime cause.

Single Herbs: Hops, Lady Slipper root, Valerian root, Passion Flower, Chamomile, Scullcap.

Combinations: Nerve Formula.

Synergistic Vitamins and Minerals: B-complex, Multi-vitamin and minerals, multi-minerals, trace minerals, Calcium, Magnesium.

KIDNEY AND BLADDER

Infection is usually the cause of kidney and bladder problems. Waste products from body processes are filtered out of the blood by the kidneys, which also regulate the fluid and electrolyte balance in the body. The wastes and excess electrolytes which are excreted, along with water, in the form of urine, are retained in the bladder until voiding. Cystitis refers to an inflammation of the bladder, whether it involves actual infection or not. Frequent, urgent and painful urination (sometimes with blood or pus) and pain in the lower abdomen and back area are symptoms of cystitis. Nephritis refers to an inflammation of the nephrons in the kidney, leading to the deterioration of that organ and sometimes death. It is nearly always a result of bacterial infection. Bright's disease refers to several extreme forms of glomerulonephritis which involves degeneration of the kidney's minute filter cells. The acute form of this disease is generally preceded by a streptococcus infection somewhere in the body and there may be no overt symptoms. However, in most cases of kidney disease, chills, fever, headache and blood or albumen (blood plasma protein) in the urine accompany the pain and tenderness in the kidney area. Kidney problems may also be indicated by edema and high blood pressure. See "Gravel and Stones" for kidney stones.

Recommended Action

Initially, one should do a juice fast, followed by a diet low in mucus and containing at least one gallon of steamdistilled or reverse osmosis water daily. Watermelon (especially its seeds) is beneficial. Potent diuretics tone and stimulate the entire urinary tract, most notably the kidneys. Remember, don't push the kidneys too hard! If there is bleeding in the urinary tract, use marshmallow, which is a specific homeostatic in this case. If it is severe, simmer one ounce marshmallow root in one pint of milk and drink a half-cup every half hour until the bleeding stops; continue taking a half-cup every hour for the rest of the day. To ensure that the organ is healing, take this remedy three times a day for the next three days. If kidney problems are complicated by, or are a result of prostate or menstrual difficulties, those problems should also be dealt with specifically at the same time.

Single Herbs: Parsley, Juniper Berries, Dandelion Root, Uva-Ursi, Gravel Root (diuretic and kidney function).

Combinations: Kidney Formula.

Synergistic Vitamins and Minerals: Carotene Vitamin A (80,000 IU daily for three months, then lowered to 20,000 IU), B6 (50 mg.), B2 (25 mg.), Choline (500 - 1000 mg.), Vitamin C (500 mg, three to six times daily), Vitamin E (200 - 1000 IU daily), Potassium (one to five grams of Potassium Chloride), Lecithin (1200 mg. twice daily).

LACTATION

Lactation is the production of milk by the female breasts, in most cases brought on by the sucking of the infant. There may be times, however, when it is necessary to take advantage of the extra assistance afforded by the galactagogue herbs which promote and enrich the flow of milk. Drinking a lot of distilled water will also help.

Single Herbs: Blessed Thistle, Marshmallow Root.

Combinations: Female Formula (two or three times daily for six weeks).

Synergistic Vitamins and Minerals: Vitamin A (20,000 IU), Vitamin D (800 IU), Multi-vitamins and minerals (one, twice daily), Calcium (250 mg. twice daily), Magnesium (125 mg. twice daily), trace minerals.

Blessed Thistle (Might Be Too Much)

When taking blessed thistle to bring in milk or just to build up supplies, start off slowly. I had one student who was going to wet nurse for a friend over a weekend. To ensure that she would have enough for both her own child and her friend's she took four capsules of blessed thistle and two cups of blessed thistle tea. Within a day she felt she was going to burst. Both babies just couldn't keep up with her production of milk.

I have also had three students who all tell the same story about how they adopted children, took blessed thistle and marshmallow tea and started producing milk within three days. All experienced a fair bit of pain in their breasts but all felt it was worth it.

LARYNGITIS

Inflammation of the larynx or voice box is known as laryngitis. It can be due to the irritation of air pollutants, emotional stress or allergic reaction but is more often the result of bacterial or viral infection or, sometimes, from just plain overwork.

Recommended Action

Mucus discharge by the inflamed membranes causes the hoarseness of laryngitis because it interferes with the normal vibration of the vocal cords. Take lemon juice and honey (equal parts either alone or mixed with water). This will relieve hoarseness while demulcent and expectorant herbs will soothe the area. The best demulcent for soothing the throat is Slippery Elm. Lozenges can be obtained in most Health Food stores.

Single Herbs: Licorice Root, Slippery Elm (for hoarseness); Ginger (for soreness); Golden Seal, Echinacea, Garlic (for infection).

Combinations: Fomentation of 3 parts Mullein and 1 part Lobelia (to the neck and throat, for soreness).

Synergistic Vitamins and Minerals: Carotene Vitamin A (30,000 IU twice daily), B-complex (two twice daily), Vitamin C (500 mg., six times daily).

LIVER AND GALL BLADDER

Gall Bladder Stones

After doing the accompanying Liver Flush you will often see hundreds of little green balls in the toilet. Some think that these are the gallstones, but they are not. They are cholesterol balls which do represent a thorough cleansing of the gall bladder and liver. Sometimes accompanying these green balls and often smaller than them are hard black or reddish coloured stones. These were probably what was giving you all the pain.

Liver and gall bladder function is essential not only to proper digestion and elimination, but also to overall body metabolism. The liver is, among other things, the body's "Master Filter", cleansing the blood of impurities and poisons, neutralizing them and transforming them into bile, an excretory fluid that has a key role as a natural laxative, intestinal alkalizer, and fat emulsifier and digestant. Bile is stored in the gall bladder until it is needed. Then it is squirted through the bile duct into the small intestine. If the bile becomes obstructed, pain and digestive disturbances result, along with a condition called jaundice. Gallstones are often responsible for this condition, which is characterized by yellow and itching skin, and yellow in the whites of the eyes, as bile salts escape into the blood and are excreted through the skin. Infection of the liver, known as hepatitis, also produces the symptoms of jaundice. Cirrhosis of the liver involves the destruction of the liver cells and their replacement by scar tissue, which gradually renders the organ unable to function and unless reversed in time, results in death. It is caused by malnutrition, fatty accumulations in the liver, and the toxic effect of excessive alcohol consumption on the liver cells. Age spots, also known as liver spots, commonly appear on exposed areas of the skin as people grow older and their livers begin to function less effectively. They seem to disappear, however, as the liver is restored to full function and the blood is cleansed. Cancers and tumors seem to be connected with an inability of the liver to carry out its normal function of neutralizing poisons and detoxifying the system.

Recommended Action

A juice fast followed by the Inner Cleanse Diet (see Appendix) is a first step to clean out and rebuild a malfunctioning liver. All processed and refined foods, as well as all chemical additives, synthetic vitamins, etc. should be strictly avoided. Hepatic and cholagogue herbs, along with a few specific liver alteratives, will stimulate and rebuild the organ. Castor oil fomentations and clay packs are excellent aids, and advantage should be taken of them. Red beets and beet juice or powder are especially beneficial, as is lemon juice, papaya juice and grape juice.

Single Herbs: Black Radish (builder, cleanser, regulator); Barberry (liver tonic); Beet powder, Dandelion, Golden Seal root, Gravel Root, Parsley (hepatics and cholagogues).

Combinations: Liver Formula (rebuilds liver); Kidney Formula (helps to strengthen liver and spleen); Lower Bowel Tonic (cleansing and detoxifying); Cleansing Formula (detoxifies).

Synergistic Vitamins and Minerals: Vitamin A (20,000 to 40,000 IU), B-Complex (high potency), B6 (50 mg.), B12 (50 mcg.), Niacin (100 mg.), Vitamin C (2,000 to 4,000 mg.), Vitamin E (400 IU), Lecithin (9,600 mg.).

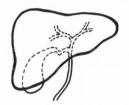

LIVER and
GALL BLADDER

Suggested Program:

If the liver is not in an acute state, use liver flush after the three day cleansing program (see Appendix).

Breakfast 2 Liver formula
Vitamin A (20,000 IU)
B Complex (high potency)
Choline (2 grams)
Vitamin C (500 mg.)
Lecithin (2,400 mg.)
Niacin (100 mg.)

Snack   Vitamin C (500 mg.)
Lecithin (1200 mg.)

Lunch   Vitamin C (500 mg.)
Vitamin E (400 IU)

Snack	Vitamin C (500 mg.) Lecithin (2,400 mg.)
Dinner	Same as Breakfast

LOW BLOOD PRESSURE

Low Blood Pressure or Hypotension, can be a sign of a long and healthy life. On the other hand, if it is accompanied by fainting, dizziness, anemia, bleeding or excessive fatigue, it may be a symptom of tuberculosis, cancer, low blood sugar, rheumatism, or adrenal, thyroid, or pituitary insufficiency.

Recommended Action

If hypotension is symptomatic of another disorder, that condition will need to be resolved first, or at least simultaneously. The best tonic for low blood pressure is regular exercise and lots of deep breathing. Herbal aids include mainly blood cleansers and builders.

Single Herbs: Beet Powder, Dandelion, Garlic, Ginseng, Sassafras, Cayenne.

LUNGS

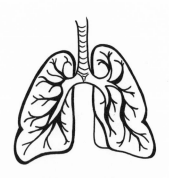

THE LUNGS

The lungs provide oxygen to the bloodstream and expel the waste carbon dioxide. Body temperature is also partly maintained by the process of respiration. Asthma and bronchitis (dealt with in detail elsewhere) are conditions which interfere with this process. Bronchitis, which is characterized by difficult breathing along with coughing, wheezing and the spitting up of mucus, is an inflammation of the bronchial tubes (air passages of the lungs). It can be acute (almost always a complication of an upper respiratory infection) or chronic (usually a result of smoking, air pollution, or a symptom of a more severe problem such as emphysema). Emphysema involves structural damage to the alveoli (tiny exchange mechanisms which are designed to get oxygen into the blood). A more or less constant sensation of suffocation comes from inhalation, followed by the inability to exhale. In pneumonia the tiny air sacs (alveoli) become filled with fluid, usually as a result of bacterial or viral infection. The body responds with inflammation and the generation of fluids which interfere with oxygen intake. Pleurisy, usually a complication of other inflammatory conditions, is infection of the sac-like membrane surrounding the lungs and pleural cavity. This causes pus, other fluids and sometimes fibrous material to be exuded into the chest cavity.

Recommended Action

The bowels must be kept free and moving in order to detoxify the system, and a liquid diet should be adhered to. The appropriate herbs should be used to keep the bacterial and viral infections under control. Congestion of the chest and lungs can be effectively relieved by the use of poultices (such as mustard packs), fomentations, clay packs, etc., while demulcent and expectorant herbs soothe the inflamed membranes and aid in expelling the mucous secretions.

Single Herbs: Slippery Elm, Licorice Root, Marshmallow Root, Mullein, Comfrey (demulcent and expectorant); Golden Seal, Garlic, Echinacea, Myrrh Gum (antiseptic).

Combinations: Lung Formula.

Synergistic Vitamins and Minerals: Carotene Vitamin A (20,000 IU twice daily), Vitamin C (500 mg., six times daily). Multi-vitamin and mineral.

LYMPHATIC SYSTEM

One of the body's major lines of defence against infection, this one-way system pulls fluids, plasma protein and other matter from the intercellular spaces into its capillaries, which are found virtually everywhere in the body. This lymph flows from the capillaries into progressively larger lymphatic vessels, passing periodically through small filters called lymph nodes - the familar "glands" that get so swollen and tender when infection is present in the body. Their normal function is to neutralize and eliminate any poisons or infectious microbes that may be present. However, during acute infection they can become overworked, swollen and sore. If the lymphatic system isn't functioning up to par, it may lose the battle and the nodes themselves become the centers of infection.

A sluggish lymphatic system which no longer effectively fulfills its function is quite possibly responsible for the resulting waste retention. Down the road this might lead to an accumulation of toxins resulting in gout, arthritis, or even cancer, heart disease and other "degenerative" diseases.

Recommended Action

Deep breathing and aerobic exercise, the best tonics for a sluggish lymphatic system, will help it to pump more effectively. Vigorous massage and bouncing on a rebounder can also stimulate it. Using a fomentation of 3 parts Mullein and 1 part Lobelia for swollen glands and drinking a tea of the same will often help. Most kidney teas will help take the stress off the lymphatic system when drunk cool to cold. Taken hot they can be used to actively cleanse the system.

Single Herbs: Mullein (specific for glands); Golden Seal, Echinacea, Myrrh Gum, Plantain (infection fighters).

Combinations: Cleansing formula, three parts Mullein with one part Lobelia, Kidney Formula.

Synergistic Vitamins and Minerals: Carotene Vitamin A (10,000 IU twice daily), B6 (75 mg.), Vitamin E (200 - 400 IU), multi-vitamin and mineral, all twelve tissue salts (especially Nat. Mur.).

MEASLES

The major characteristic of this contagious disease is a reddish skin rash which is common to both of its two forms. The first, Rubella ("German" or "Three-day" measles), has a light pink rash that fades in three or four days and does not peel; it sometimes doesn't even appear. The symptoms, such as head cold and cough, are mild and the fever is not too high. The glands behind the ears usually swell and there may be pain in the joints for about a week.

The second, Rubeola ("Common" or "Seven-day" measles), is more serious and more likely to involve complications. It is characterized by fever, cough, inflammation of the eyes and tiny red patches (with white crystal-like centers) inside the cheeks and mouth. These last are definite indications of Rubeola and are called Koplik's spots. The rash, which eventually peels, appears a few days later as small red spots surrounded by darker red patches that run together forming irregular blotches. Complications can result, such as a cough that leads to laryngitis, bronchitis or pneumonia, ear or eye infections, heart problems or inflammation of the brain (encephalitis).

Recommended Action

Take nothing but juices, distilled or reverse osmosis water and herb teas for the first few days. Keep the bowels free and moving by using Lower Bowel Tonic and/or garlic or catnip enemas. Temporary relief can be achieved by the use of Saffron, which will help the rash to break out and alleviate the fever. Use Golden Seal or Apple Cider Vinegar to relieve itching of the skin. Use diaphoretic and nervine teas to help maintain the elimination of toxins through the skin and to soothe a system weary from inflammation, irritation and itching.

Single Herbs: Yarrow, Chamomile, Geranium, Saffron, Eyebright, Red Raspberry leaves, Golden Seal (cleansing and diaphoretic); Siberian Ginseng.

Synergistic Vitamins and Minerals: During convalescence: Carotene Vitamin A (20,000 IU twice daily), Vitamin C (500 mg. twice daily), Vitamin E 400 IU.

MEMORY

The cerebral cortex of the brain controls memory function. Arteriosclerosis in the arteries leading to the brain, along with inorganic mineral deposits in the brain cells themselves, results in ischemia (cell starvation from lack of oxygen and nutrients). This interferes with the thinking processes and produces what is usually recognized as senile behaviour.

Recommended Action

Drink large amounts of steam-distilled or reverse osmosis water to leach out the inorganic deposits. Ensure that the brain receives proper nourishment to rebuild the deteriorating cells. Maintain and promote good circulation.

Single Herbs: Blue Vervain, Gotu Kola, Fo-ti-teng, Blessed Thistle (specifics for the brain).

Synergistic Vitamins and Minerals: Vitamin B formula (two, twice daily), Vitamin C (500 mg. three times daily), Glutamine, Tyrosine, Lecithin (1200 mg. twice daily).

Gotu Kola For Memory

Probably the best herb for memory is Gotu Kola. It has the ability to aid both circulation and the oxygen content of the blood circulating to the brain, thus stimulating the metabolism of protein to start the memory process.

MENOPAUSE

Menopause is the cessation of menses when the uterus shrinks and the ovaries quit producing stimulating hormones. Irregular menses accompanied by "hot flashes", headaches, insomnia and general irritability often precede cessation by a few months to several years. The changes in body chemistry brought on by the reduction of certain female hormones cause these symptoms.

Diminished interest in sex is often associated with menopause but is not necessarily always the case. A woman's sexual activity can often be stimulated by the diminished possibility of pregnancy.

Single Herbs: Dong Quai (Hormone regulator), Black Cohosh, Blue Cohosh, Blessed Thistle, Siberian Ginseng.

Combinations: Female Formula.

Synergistic Vitamins and Minerals: Vitamin A (20,000 to 40,000 IU), B-Complex, B6 (25 - 100 mg.), B1 (50 mg.), PABA (up to 100 mg., a precursor for estrogen), Pantothenic acid (up to 100 mg., helps to delay menopause), Vitamin C (500 mg. three times daily), Vitamin E (800 - 1,200 IU) stimulates production of estrogen, Calcium/Magnesium plus D (2 tablets twice daily for rest of life).

Menopause

Mrs. H. came in with a problem of 'hot sweats' from her change of life. While she was sitting in front of me she started having a sweating session which completely soaked through her wool suit. She had a pretty bad case, so she took two Female formula three times daily and two Dong Quai. Within six weeks she was symptom-free.

MENSTRUATION

Menstruation is the term for the discharge from the uterus of blood and other materials essential for pregnancy because fertilization has not occurred. Cramps, nervous tension, backache, water retention, menorrhagia (excessive or profuse flow), amenorrhea (suppressed or stopped flow) or dysmenorrhea (painful flow) are common menstrual difficulties.

Recommended Action

Emmenagogue herbs stimulate and promote normal menstrual function and flow. If congestion from a recent cold is the cause of amenorrhea or dysmenorrhea, a good diaphoretic may be all that is necessary to relieve the problem. Tonics should be used in addition to stimulating diaphoretics if systemic or specific (organ) weakness is the cause. Avoid the use of purgative and strong cathartic laxatives.

Diet can also be a major cause of menstrual difficulties and can therefore correct some problems. The diet should include whole grains, nuts and seeds (especially sprouted), fresh fruits and vegetables, almonds, buckwheat, millet, oats, sesame and sunflower seeds (rich in Vitamin E and B-complex), blackstrap molasses, grapes, and red beets (rich in iron). Yogurt, miso, sauerkraut and other fermented foods which contain Vitamin B-12 help to restore the normal menstrual function. Thyroid deficiency may be indicated by irregular or profuse menstruation (see "Thyroid"). Lack of Calcium and Magnesium is also a common major cause of cramps.

Single Herbs: Ginger, White Oak Bark, Yarrow (orally or as a douche, for

Relief from Menstrual Cramps

On the inside of the leg, four finger widths up from the ankle bone is an accupressure point which, when stimulated forcefully for about five minutes will often relieve menstrual cramps.

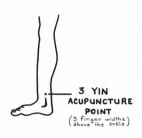

3 YIN
ACUPUNCTURE
POINT
(3 finger widths above the ankle)

menorrhagia); Black Cohosh, Blue Cohosh, Chamomile, Squaw Vine, St. Johns Wort (amenorrhea); Ginger, Pennyroyal, Squaw Vine (dysmenorrhea).

Combinations: Female Formula.

Synergistic Vitamins and Minerals: B-complex, B6 (25 - 75 mg.), Vitamin C (500 - 3000 mg. daily), Multi-minerals, Calcium (500 mg. daily), Magnesium (250 mg. daily), tissue salt Mag Phos 6x.

MUCUS

Mucus (noun) is a thick fluid which lubricates and protects the surfaces of the mucous (adjective) membranes by which it is secreted. Most people are familiar with the presence of mucus in the passages of the upper respiratory tract, nose and throat, but it is also present throughout the gastrointestinal and urogenital tracts.

Phlegm is the term for mucus in the throat, chest and lungs. A certain amount of mucus is vital to the function of body systems, but excessive secretion clogs the system, leads to degenerative disease and provides a potential haven for germs (see Infection). There is a possibility that excess mucus is produced by a shortage of potassium chloride (the compound in the blood that keeps fibrin in solution preventing it from coagulating) causes excess mucus production.

Recommended Action

A few days of juice fasting will help to clean out the excess mucus. Then adopt a diet low in mucus by cutting down on dairy products, refined carbohydrates and meats. Eat fresh fruits, vegetables and potassium (vegetable) broth to obtain that element. Expectorant herbs are also beneficial in expelling mucus from the respiratory tract.

Single Herbs: Elderberry Extract (potassium); Comfrey, Fenugreek, Licorice, Marshmallow, Mullein, Thyme (expectorants); Lobelia Extract (emetic expectorant: phlegm is expelled in vomiting); Golden Seal root (controls quality and quantity of mucus).

Combinations: Cleansing Formula, Lung Formula, Stomach Formula, Lower Bowel Tonic.

Synergistic Vitamins and Minerals: Carotene Vitamin A (20,00 IU twice daily), Vitamin C (500 mg., six times daily), multi-tissue salts.

MUSCLE STRAIN OR SORENESS

Overexertion, or working muscles harder or longer than they are accustomed to, is the most common cause of muscle strain or soreness. Lactic acid is a byproduct of the chemical release of energy, which builds up in the cells of the muscle causing soreness, fatigue and stiffness.

Recommended Action

Proper diet and adequate exercise will maintain muscle tone and prevent soreness in normal circumstances. Calcium and magnesium supplements help as they are essential to muscle function. Massage relaxes the muscle fibers and helps to move lactic acid out of the cells and is therefore excellent for soreness and stiffness. It is more effective if herbal liniments are used.

Single Herbs: Siberian Ginseng, Kava Kava (relaxing); Arnica Tincture, Cayenne Tincture (liniment for pain and swelling); Wormwood, Witch Hazel, Lobelia Extract (liniments); Alfalfa, Dandelion Root (calcium and magnesium); Saffron (prevents excess buildup of lactic acid).

Combinations: Muscle Relaxing Formula, Nerve Formula.

Synergistic Vitamins and Minerals: Carotene Vitamin A (two - 10,000 IU twice daily), B-complex, B15 (100 mg. twice daily), Calcium and Magnesium (500/250 mg. daily), Multi-minerals (two twice daily), Lecithin (12,000 mg. twice daily).

Soothing Liniment

A good liniment for sore muscles, bursitis, bruises, pulled muscles and the like can be made from equal parts of Arnica Tincture and Cayenne Tincture. To these a little birch oil can be added if available. Rub the liniment into the area and relax.

NAUSEA

Nausea, which can be caused by vertigo, morning sickness, food poisoning, emotional disturbance, improper eating and bacterial infections (especially of the intestinal tract), refers to the sensation that one is about to vomit.

Recommended Action

Anti-emetic herbs will generally relieve nausea unless it is caused by an acute case of food poisoning or infection. The cause is often the presence of putrid or undigested matter in the stomach, in which case it is best to cleanse the stomach by using an emetic to induce vomiting. If the emetic is preceded by a stimulant such as Cayenne, Peppermint or Elder, this will prevent undue strain on the body from the "upward purge".

Single Herbs: Lobelia Extract (3 - 5 drops) Meadow Sweet, Cloves, Catnip, Peppermint, Spearmint, Peach Leaves, Red Raspberry Leaves (anti-emetic).

The following, in large amounts, cause Emesis: Lobelia Extract, Cayenne and Bayberry, Blessed Thistle, Dry Mustard (emetics).

Combinations: Acute:"Po Chai". Chronic: Stomach Formula, Digest, Lower Bowel Tonic.

Synergistic Vitamins and Minerals: Calcium/Magnesium (500/250 mg.), multi-tissue salts.

NERVOUS DISORDERS

Afflictions of the brain and spinal cord and problems in the peripheral nervous system are classed as nervous disorders. Included in this type of problem are sclerosis, hardening of the brain or spinal cord tissues and various types of palsy. Multiple sclerosis is related to the brain and spinal cord and involves little patches of hardened or deadened tissue. It is called lateral sclerosis if it affects only the side portions of the spinal cord and posterolateral sclerosis if it affects both the back and side portions. Depending on the body parts which are connected with the affected nervous tissue, vision, speech or other body functions may be impaired. Palsy is either temporary or permanent partial paralysis. In Bell's palsy usually just one side of the face is affected. In Cerebral palsy, brain damage, which usually occurs prior to or during birth, causes muscular coordination problems. In Parkinson's disease, also known as shaking palsy or paralysis agitans, certain cells in the brain's muscle coordination center deteriorate.

Recommended Action

In advanced cases of nerve disorder, often little can be done, but if nothing is tried little gain can be expected. To eliminate toxic wastes from damaged and degenerating nervous tissue, cleanse the bowel and the blood and adopt a diet low in mucus. Nervine and antispasmodic herbs are essential for regenerating and renewing the nervous system. Cayenne, which has antispasmodic qualities and is a powerful circulatory stimulant and nutritive tonic, has alone been known to resolve some cases of temporary paralysis. Calcium and magnesium, principal ingredients of the myelin sheath which surrounds the nerves and nerve cells, can be found in plentiful supply in Alfalfa. A few drops of garlic oil followed by B and B tincture drops in the ear, will be beneficial in helping to rebuild the motor nerve centers at the base of the brain. Oil of Evening Primrose can help to build the myelin sheath.

Single Herbs: Oil of Evening Primrose, Alfalfa, Cayenne (nerve nutrients); Black Cohosh, Blue Cohosh, Blue Vervain, Gotu Kola (specifics for the brain); Scullcap (specific for spinal cord); Lobelia Extract, Hops, Valerian, Wood Betony (nervine tonics and antispasmodics).

Combinations: Nerve Formula, Muscle Relaxant Formula, Cleansing Formula (cleansing), B and B tincture, Lower Bowel Tonic (constipation).

Synergistic Vitamins and Minerals: B-complex (two twice daily), Vitamin C (500 mg. twice daily), Multi-mineral (two twice daily), Trace Minerals, multi-tissue salts, Lecithin (1200 mg. twice daily).

NERVOUS TENSION

Nervous Tension

There is hardly anyone who doesn't suffer from time to time from a little nervous tension in our modern world. The cases come in daily. Nervous tension can cause a multitude of other problems as well. The following is a program we gave Mr. J., who came in with a fairly bad case of 'nerves' from business and domestic stresses. He was given two B-complex twice daily, two Adrenal complex twice daily, One C-complex four times daily, Calcium Magnesium plus D four daily, and two multiminerals twice daily. He also eliminated as much of his stress as possible by working fewer hours, thus helping both the business and domestic problems, and by starting a relaxing hobby. Within three months the tensions were much less; in six months the supplements were cut in half. Now, two years later, Mr. J. takes one B-complex daily and considers life 'clear sailing'.

Nervous tension is characterized by restlessness, mental and physical unrest, emotional agitation, tension or tightness of the nerves and muscles, or a state of non-specific nervous excitation. The muscle tension causes headaches, stomach upset, muscle soreness and strain especially in the neck and shoulder area. Nervous tension is not actually a disorder, but a neuromuscular reaction to anxiety, stress or emotional conflict (either conscious or unconscious). This condition requires much greater amounts of calcium, magnesium, B vitamins and other specific nutrients for the body. If these nutrients are leached out of the body by excessive consumption of sugar and refined carbohydrates or if they are lacking in the diet, they will be taken from other sources within the body. Consequently, blood vessels, bones and especially nerves and the nerve sheaths suffer in an attempt to satisfy the body's metabolic need for calcium. The result is that the nerves, which have become frayed like exposed electrical wires, spark or short-circuit where they cross or travel in proximity.

Recommended Action

All refined sugars and starches should be eliminated from the diet, which should be supplemented with organic calcium, magnesium, Vitamin C and B-complex. Nervine herbs are good for rebuilding weakened and frayed nerves and nerve sheaths. Often adrenal complex is very useful to reduce stress.

Single Herbs: Alfalfa, Comfrey (Magnesium, Calcium); Hops (sedative nervine); Valerian, Lobelia Extract, Black Cohosh, Blue Cohosh, Lady Slipper root, Kava Kava (relaxant Nervines).

Combinations: Muscle Relaxant Formula, Nerve Formula.

Synergistic Vitamins and Minerals: Vitamin A (10,000 IU daily), B-complex (two twice daily), Vitamin C (500 mg. three times daily), Vitamin D (400 IU daily), Calcium/Magnesium (600/300 mg. daily), Multi-minerals, Trace minerals, Raw adrenal gland (when associated with stress).

NOSEBLEED

Nosebleed (clinically known as epistaxis) is a common problem and often results from physical injury, such as a blow to the nose. Excessive dryness, sudden change in atmospheric pressure, scratching with the fingernail or blowing the nose too forcefully can also cause injury to the nasal lining. High blood pressure, nasal polyps or tumors, a blood disorder or simply a calcium deficiency (leaves nasal blood vessels weak and susceptible to rupture) may be indicated by persistent or recurring nosebleeds.

Recommended Action

Usually drinking a teaspoon of Cayenne in a glass of warm water will remedy a nosebleed. In severe cases snuff Golden Seal or White Oak Bark tea up the nose; their astringent and homeostatic properties suffice to stop the bleeding. Bayberry bark and White Oak bark are astringents and should be taken into the nose daily for recurrent cases (especially where polyps are present). These will strengthen the blood vessels and tissues of the nasal passages. Either use them as a tea and inhale through the nose or spray them in with an atomizer; or by using a straw, carefully inhale a very small amount of powder up the nose. Taking a calcium supplement will help to strengthen the nasal blood vessels.

Single Herbs: Cayenne (vulnerary, hemostatic); Golden Seal root, White Oak bark, Barberry bark, Yarrow (hemostatic and astringent).

Synergistic Vitamins and Minerals: Vitamin C (500 mg. four to six times daily), Bioflavenoids (1000 - 2000 mg. daily), Calcium/Magnesium (500/250 mg. daily), Multi-vitamins and minerals (one twice daily).

OBESITY

See Weight Loss.

PANCREAS

The pancreas, a small gland which lies behind the stomach, has a twofold purpose. It functions as part of the digestive system by secreting a powerful enzymatic juice through the pancreatic ducts into the small intestine. It also functions as part of the endocrine (ductless gland) system by secreting insulin and glucagon directly into the bloodstream. These substances regulate the body's use of glucose and therefore its blood sugar level. In Diabetes mellitus (also called hyperglycemia) the body cells are unable to metabolize or use glucose due to the insufficiency or unavailability of insulin. Consequently, the glucose must remain in the bloodstream. In hyperglycemia (too much sugar in the blood) the body will try to eliminate some of this excess sugar through the kidneys. Normally they operate to prevent glucose from being lost in the urine. Water and salts are lost under this abnormal condition and it may lead to dehydration. If diabetes is severe and untreated, metabolizing fats and proteins instead of carbohydrates causes excessive amounts of keto acids (byproducts of fat metabolism) in the blood and urine. Hypoglycemia (not enough sugar in the blood) can involve the pancreas or the adrenal glands (see also Hypoglycemia). Treatment of the diabetic should only be done under the guidance of a Health Practitioner.

Recommended Action

To prevent dehydration, drink a gallon of steam-distilled or reverse osmosis water daily. This will also benefit the blood and urine. When drinking fruit juices ensure that each mouthful is swished around in the mouth for at least 15 seconds, to mix in the saliva well and break down the fruit sugars. Also fruits and vegetables should be well chewed and all concentrated or refined starches and sugars eliminated from the diet.

Single Herbs: Cedar Berries (strengthens endocrine function), Fringe Tree Bark (strengthens digestive function).

Combinations: Glucose Formula.

Synergistic Vitamins and Minerals: B-complex (two twice daily), Vitamin C (500 mg. six times daily), Vitamin E (400 IU), Multi-vitamin and mineral (one twice daily), zinc, chromium, lecithin, nucleic acid.

PARASITES

Parasites (either plant or animal) are organisms that take their nourishment from the host in which (or on which) they are living. Pathogens are parasites which cause damage and disease. Viruses, bacteria, rickettsia, fungi and worms are all parasites affecting man. Most people are familiar with viral and bacterial infections (see Infection). Typhus Q and Rocky Mountain Spotted Fever are caused by rickettsia, transmitted by fleas and ticks. Fungal diseases are caused by moulds and yeasts. They do not produce chlorophyll and must get their food from other organic matter. Ringworm, athlete's foot, yeast infections, candidiasis or moniliasis of the skin, mouth and vagina are all superficial fungus infections; coccidioicomycis ("Cocci") and histoplasmosis, which attack the organs of the body, are deep systemic-type fungal infections. Parasitic worms

PANCREAS

are roundworms (nematodes) including pinworms. hookworms and trichina or flatworms including tapeworms and flukes. Parasites are the cause of a variety of symptoms, such as fever, chills, nausea, diarrhea, skin rashes, itching and breathing difficulties, and may be responsible for allergic reactions, lesions, abnormal growths and toxic reactions similar to poisoning. Nutritional loss, anemia, cell damage, trauma and obstructions in organs and body systems are caused particularly by worms, their presence being indicated by restlessness at night, excessive nose picking, grinding the teeth and rectal itching.

Recommended Action

Although improper hygiene and sanitation habits are usually related to worms, internal uncleanliness is the major cause, since all parasites function essentially as scavengers in the overall ecological system. Virtually all parasitic organisms operate in the same way as germs, acting as "garbagemen" to clean up the environment. It is important to cleanse and tone the bowel, blood and liver, the last often being the first organ subject to parasitic attack. Enemas involving astringent and anthelmintic herbs are beneficial. Anthelmintic herbs are of two types - vermifuges (expel worms) and vermicides (destroy worms). Better results will be achieved if these are taken with a diet low in mucus and one including foods such as onions, garlic, pickles and large quantities of pumpkin seed, all of which are offensive to worms. Black Walnut Extract preceded by a few drops of garlic oil is a potent fungicide. (It is also a specific remedy for persistent yeast-related diaper rash). Since superficial fungus infections thrive on warm moisture, make sure that the area is kept cool and dry. Remember that parasites are everywhere and the only way to avoid them is through internal and external cleanliness. We have a natural internal barrier against parasites, being HCl in the stomach. Adequate acid formation in the stomach will destroy most parasites.

Single Herbs: Chamomile, Chapparal, Garlic, Peach Leaves, Male Fern, Wormwood, Black Walnut, Senna, Pumpkin Seeds (anthelmintic); Black Walnut Extract, Garlic (vermicide and fungicide).

Combinations: Lower Bowel Tonic, Liver Formula.

Getting Rid of Those Worms

Parasites are everywhere. Dr. J. R. Christopher used to say that a small proportion of his patients over 45 yrs had parasites - 95%! The best herbs for parasites that we have found are Wormwood and Male Fern root. We also suggest taking lots of garlic and pumpkin seeds in your diet. The best time to work on parasites is three days before the full moon till four days after the full moon. Many parasites lay their eggs at this time and are therefore the most vulnerable.

PERIODONTAL DISEASE

Periodontal means "located around a tooth", and may refer to any disorder of the gums or other supporting structures of the teeth. Gingivitis (inflammation

Periodontal Problems and Minerals

Periodontal problems plague more people over 35 than any other disease. This can be traced back to their dietary habits. It has been shown in many studies that most Periodontal problems can be aided with minerals, especially Calcium, Magnesium, and Potassium. We suggest 1000 mg. of both Potassium and Calcium daily with 500 mg. of Magnesium. A good multi-mineral and trace mineral is also necessary. As far as herbs go, we suggest Oak Bark, Myrrh, and Propolis. All are useful powders to place (against the gums) in the mouth before going to bed. The above very simple program has aided many a person.

of the gums) is the most common form of periodontal disease and is frequently a result of improper diet, ill-fitting dentures, uneven bite, plaque buildup or some other source of irritation. In necrotizing gingivitis (trench mouth) infection is the cause. Pyorrhea (periodontitis) is a condition resulting from the above if the inflamed gums (which are swollen and red, and bleed when brushed) are not cared for. It is characterized by receding gums, weakened tooth sockets and loose teeth. Thrush is a yeast infection of the mouth, characterized by creamy white patches coating the inside of the mouth, and is generally accompanied by a foul odour. If it gets into the bronchial tubes and lungs it can be fatal.

Recommended Action

Use organic calcium supplements to strengthen the teeth and tooth sockets along with astringent herbs to tone and restore life to the gums.

Single Herbs: Red Raspberry Leaf tea and White Oak Bark (applied between cheek and gums morning and night for all cases); Black Walnut extract (antibiotic and antifungal), for trench mouth and thrush, Golden Seal root.

Synergistic Vitamins and Minerals: Carotene Vitamin A (20,000 IU), B-complex (one twice daily), Vitamin C (500 mg. six times daily), Vitamin D (800 IU daily), Calcium/ Magnesium (600/300 mg.), Potassium (600 mg.), Multi-mineral, trace mineral.

PITUITARY

The pituitary governs the other endocrine and reproductive glands in the system and is therefore often referred to as the "master gland" of the body. Metabolic processes (such as growth) and the maintenance of proper fluid levels in the body are also regulated by the pituitary gland. A multitude of problems such as abnormal growth patterns and disorders of the thyroid, adrenals, kidneys and reproductive organs can result from malfunction of the pituitary.

Single Herbs: Alfalfa, Kelp, Ginseng, Gotu Kola, Fo-ti-teng, Chlorophyll.

Synergistic Vitamins and Minerals: B-complex, Choline, Niacin, Vitamin C (500 mg. six times daily), Multi-vitamin and mineral, Calcium (250 mg.), Magnesium (500 mg.), Raw Pituitary.

PROSTATE

The most common problem of the male genito·urinary tract relates to this gland, which is an accessory male sex organ. It is situated directly beneath the bladder and is shaped somewhat like a donut, it encircles the urethra (the urinary outlet). Its purpose is to contract and squeeze its fluid secretions (containing elements necessary to the semen) into the urethral tract during ejaculation. Prostatitus, or inflammation and enlargement, can partially or totally block the flow of urine out of the bladder, resulting in urine retention. This causes the bladder to become distended, weak and susceptible to infection as a result of the increased amount of bacteria in the retained urine. Infection is easily transmitted from the bladder up the ureters to the kidneys. Benign or cancerous tumors, the formation of stones (calculi), hardening (sclerosis) and congestion (from prolonged stimulation followed by suppression or incomplete ejaculation) can also afflict the prostate. Frequent and increased urination (especially at night), difficulty in urinating, lessening of the force of flow and an accompanying burning sensation are all symptoms of prostate problems.

Recommended Action

Incorporate raw seeds (especially pumpkin seeds), nuts and whole grains into the diet to obtain elements such as zinc and Vitamin F (essential fatty acids) which are important for prostate health. Raw pumpkin seeds eaten daily are helpful for almost all prostate troubles. Juice and distilled or reverse osmosis water should be taken in large amounts; in all cases juice fasting is also very effective. All diuretic herbs, specifically Parsley and Buchu, have a tonic effect on the genito·urinary tract and are helpful for this condition.

Single Herbs: Chaparral, Echinacea (cleansers, alterative tonics); Golden Seal (diuretic and antiseptic); Juniper Berries, Parsley, Uva-Ursi, Buchu (diuretics and tonics for urinary tract); Ginseng (specific for male reproductive organs).

Combinations: Kidney Formula.

Synergistic Vitamins and Minerals: Vitamin A (20,000 IU), B-6 (50 mg.), Vitamin C (500 mg. three to six times daily), Vitamin E (400-1200 IU), Zinc (75 mg.), Copper (5 mg.), Multiminerals, Bee Pollen, Lecithin, Fish liver oil.

RHEUMATIC FEVER

Streptococcus infections such as strep throat or scarlet fever precede rheumatic fever, which may affect the skin, bones and joints and causes symptoms resembling arthritis or other connective tissue disorders. Sydenhams Chorea or St. Vitus' Dance (a spasmodic twitching of the body) occurs when the brain and spinal cord are affected. Even without these other symptoms it frequently causes carditis, an inflammation of the heart. This in turn can cause permanent damage (rheumatic heart disease) to the heart valves or to the muscles of the interior lining. Aching in different joints, abnormal rhythm of the heart, small lumps or nodules under the skin, rash, fatigue, fever, and loss of weight or appetite are all indicative of rheumatic fever.

Recommended Action

Juice fasting will cleanse the entire system, while Lower Bowel Tonic or garlic and/or a Catnip enema will keep the bowels free and moving. The individual symptoms should be dealt with separately as indicated under nervous disorders, arthritis, heart problems, etc., and be careful not to overwork the heart. There have been indications that the bioflavinoids (Vitamin P - citrin, hesperedin, rutin, etc.) have an advantageous affect on rheumatic fever. See also: Fevers, Scarlet Fever. The Arthritis diet (in appendix) should be adopted.

SCARLET FEVER

Scarlet Fever, also known as "Scarlatina" (in its milder form), is an acute streptococcus infection. It usually begins with a sore throat, swollen lymph nodes and a phlegmatic cough and is indicated by a scarlet skin rash, particularly in the groin and armpits, and by a red coating on the tongue ("Strawberry tongue"). The rash begins to show when the infection has spread throughout the system and is frequently accompanied by fever, chills, vomiting and, in some cases, convulsions. The rash will clear and the other symptoms subside within a few days, but the body is left in a weakened condition and is susceptible to other bacterial infections or to further complications such as rheumatic fever or rheumatic heart disease. Care should therefore be taken to prevent further complications of the strep infection.

Nip Scarlet Fever in The Bud

Scarlet Fever in itself is not a really a severe problem, but the complications that can arise from it are. It can do severe damage to both the heart and the kidneys. Scarlet Fever often affects young children whose parents have had strep throat. The parents, trying to follow a 'Natural Way', often get confused and try to fix the strep throat with Vitamin C and Vitamin A which are not strong enough. If the strep throat is passed to the child, it is probable that Scarlet Fever will result in the child. If the parents would take antibiotics for their throat problem, spending the next three to six months cleaning up the side effects of the antibiotics, the results would be a lot better than spending years trying to fix the child's weakened kidneys or heart from the Scarlet Fever.

Recommended Action

Do a few days of juice fasting along with plenty of Lower Bowel Tonic or Catnip or Garlic enemas which will keep the bowels free and moving. Take copious amounts of liquid every hour, if possible, while taking Saffron (especially in combination with Catnip). This will help to bring out the rash and often has the added effect of bringing down the fever. To draw out the toxins use ginger baths and diaphoretic herbs and drink lots of fluids to replace those lost. Infection fighting herbs should also be used to regulate this condition. As Scarlet Fever can be severe in some cases, detroying the kidneys and weaking the heart, a physician should be consulted. It is often more prudent to take an antibiotic to get over this problem easily and spend the next few months rebuilding the body from the effects of the antibiotic than it is to spend many years rebuilding a damaged heart or kidneys!

Single Herbs: Catnip (for enemas, also orally as a diaphoretic and febrifuge); Garlic (for enemas, also orally as antibiotic); Saffron (diaphoretic, encourages break out of rash); Ginger, Yarrow, Blessed Thistle, Sage (diaphoretics); Golden Seal, Echinacea.

Combinations: Lower Bowel Tonic (to keep bowel free and moving).

SHINGLES

In this condition herpes zoster virus (thought to be similar to the chicken pox virus) causes infection of the peripheral nerves of the body. Swelling of the lymph nodes, reddening of the skin and eruption of blisters are indications of shingles. The blisters are extremely sensitive to the touch and may itch or burn, but within a few weeks they dry up, crust over and finally drop off. There are usually no serious long-range effects unless the eyes become infected, in which case blindness may result. This condition is sometimes followed by temporary paralysis or neuralgia of the affected area.

Recommended Action

A three-day juice fast along with plenty of Lower Bowel Tonic will cleanse the system of toxins. Nervine herbs, particularly the nerve tonic, will soothe and strengthen the inflamed nerves, while calcium and magnesium supplements will help rebuild them. Apple cider vinegar diluted with water, used as often as necessary to bathe the affected areas of the skin, will give temporary relief. Castor oil and fomentations of the glandular combination are also good used this way but have a better effect on swollen lymph nodes.

Single Herbs: Valerian, Hops (calm the nerves).

Combinations: Nerve Formula.

SHOCK

During shock the protective reflexes and vital processes of the body (particularly the blood pressure and circulation) become dangerously depressed. The trauma of serious injury, the sudden spread of severe infection, a great loss of blood, a serious allergic reaction or a severe emotional trauma may bring on shock. It is characterized by pale skin colour and cold, moist skin. Other indications are dilated pupils, a vacant look, shallow and irregular breathing and a weak but fast pulse.

Shock

Shock is a fairly normal reaction to any dramatic situation, be it an accident, severe loss of blood or emotional trauma. In cases of shock always give 1/4 - 1/2 tsp. of cayenne pepper in some water if the person is conscious. If unconscious, put a few drops of Bach Rescue Remedy on the lips. Get the person to sip a glass of water with a few drops of Rescue Remedy in it if conscious. Always keep the person warm.

Recommended Action

The most important measure to normalize blood pressure and circulation is to take one teaspoon of Cayenne in a glass of warm water. Massaging Lobelia Extract into the abdominal area, the solar plexus, the neck and back of the head will relax the muscles and nerves, allowing freer circulation. Taking nervine herbs, either orally or as enemas, will relax the system even further and normalize vital processes.

Single Herbs: Cayenne, Lobelia Extract, Hops, Scullcap, Valerian, Catnip.

Combinations: Nerve Formula, Bach Rescue Remedy.

SKIN PROBLEMS

Acne (dealt with elsewhere), eczema and psoriasis are common skin problems. Eczema is characterized by blistered or crusted and scaling lesions which are almost always accompanied by severe itching. In this case secondary infection can be a problem, especially if the top layers of skin have been destroyed by scratching. Psoriasis (often a persistent and chronic problem which can last a lifetime) is characterized by pink or red patches covered with silvery scales and rarely produces pain or itching. A breakdown in the function of the skin as an eliminative organ is indicated in all skin disorders. The skin plays a major part in excreting wastes resulting from body processes and is therefore often referred to as the "third kidney" or "third lung". Poor bathing habits, using soaps that clog the pores, wearing synthetic materials which don't "breathe" and eating foods which produce excessive amounts of mucus and toxic wastes all prevent proper functioning of the skin. When any area of the skin ceases to function properly, a greater burden is placed upon the remainder which still functions effectively, resulting in congestion and deterioration as toxic wastes attempt to escape through a limited area of skin surface.

Recommended Action

A juice fast and a diet low in mucus along with herbs for the bowel and blood will cleanse the body of mucus and toxic waste. Skin irritation can be relieved by using Chickweed in the form of a fomentation or ointment, while Apple Cider Vinegar or Yellow Dock tea applied externally will relieve itching. Aloe Vera Gel may be taken internally or externally to relieve skin irritation. Black Walnut Extract, or a poultice or fomentation combination, is also beneficial. The best herb found for skin problems is Oil of Evening Primrose.

Single Herbs: Chickweed and Chickweed Ointment, Aloe Vera, Black Walnut Extract (specifics for skin); Echinacea, Burdock, Dandelion Root (blood cleansers), Oil of Evening Primrose (builder).

Combinations: Cleansing Formula, Lower Bowel Tonic.

Synergistic Vitamins and Minerals: Vitamin A (20,000 IU), B-complex (two twice daily), Niacin (125 mg. twice daily), Vitamin C (500 mg. three six times daily), Multi-vitamins and minerals.

TENDONITIS

Tendons are the elastic fibers that connect muscles to bones. When they become inflamed, usually as a result of injury or sometimes infection, the condition is known as tendonitis. Weakness of a particular muscle and specific pain associated with any movement of the muscle are indicative of tendonitis. Calcium deposits around the tendons and synovial bursa of the shoulder create a condition known as calcific tendonitis or bursitis.

Recommended Action

It is important first of all to locate and remove the source of the inflammation. Bone, Flesh and Cartilage combination used both internally and externally will not only help to heal the injury but will also relieve the inflammation in the tendon. Massaging liquid analgesic or Lobelia Extract into the affected area will give some relief from pain.

Single Herbs: Comfrey ("cell proliferant", heals damaged tissues); Cayenne/Arnica Tinctures (equal parts as a liniment).

Combinations: Muscle Relaxing Formula, Nerve Formula, B & B Tincture, Bone, Flesh and Cartilage.

Synergistic Vitamins and Minerals: Vitamin A (10,000 IU), B-complex, Vitamin C (500 mg. three times daily), Multi-minerals, Calcium/Magnesium (600/300 mg.), Potassium (300 mg.), trace minerals.

Tendonitis

Tendonitis occurs very often in musicians and athletes. The best thing we have found for this is Dr. Christopher's formula "Bone Flesh and Cartilage". You make a fomentation out of this and apply it hot at least once daily. This product is also available in ointment form which can be applied topically. The accompanying vitamins should be taken with the Muscle Relaxing Formula and Calcium Pangamate (N,N-dimethylglycine) 100mg. two times daily.

THYROID

The thyroid (a butterfly-shaped gland located just below the Adam's apple in front of the trachea or windpipe) regulates many important body processes. It combines iodine compounds in the blood with certain amino acids to secrete hormones. Basal metabolism (rate of chemical processes such as changing food into energy and building proteins), growth, thought processes, maintenance of body fluid balance, blood cholestrol levels and adequate func-

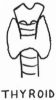

THYROID

tioning of other endocrine glands are some of the body processes which the thyroid affects. Sluggishness, absentmindedness, nervousness, weight gain and chronic fatigue indicate an underactive thyroid (hypothyroidism), while increased metabolic rate, nervousness, restlessness, weight loss and a constant feeling of being too hot and sweating indicate an overactive thyroid (hyperthyroidism). Goiter (an abnormal enlargement of the thyroid gland) is a symptom of either one of these conditions.

Single Herbs: Kelp, Dulse (specific tonics for thyroid); Mullein (specific for entire glandular system including thyroid); Alfalfa (specific for pituitary which regulates the thyroid); Garlic, Cayenne (antiatherosclerotics, assist cholesterol function of thyroid); Parsley (diuretic assists body fluid balance function of thyroid).

TONSILLITIS

The palatine or faucial tonsils (located on either side of the inner throat, behind the tongue) work together with the pharyngeal tonsil (located in the nasopharynx or upper part of the throat) to form the body's front line of defense against airborne bacteria entering the body through the mouth and nose. They are part of the lymphatic system, and when they become inflamed, from fighting infection, the condition is known as tonsillitis.

Recommended Action

Acute tonsillitis (a sudden bacterial invasion of the nose and throat) can be remedied by a three-day juice fast along with herbs that cleanse and strengthen the glandular system and those that keep the bowel free and moving. A toxic condition that the lymphatic system is unable to throw off is indicated in chronic tonsillitis, and long-term measures are necessary to clean and tone the bowel, the blood and the lymphatic system. In the abscessed condition known as quinsy, gargling with an astringent as well as a tea made of three parts Mullein, one part Lobelia (1 tsp of combined herbs in a cup of boiled water) may be an urgent necessity along with the same treatment as indicated for chronic tonsillitis. You have to be patient with tonsillitis and get plenty of bed rest!

Single Herbs: Golden Seal, Echinacea (infection fighters); Mullein (specific for glandular system); Bayberry (astringent gargle).

Synergistic Vitamins and Minerals: Carotene Vitamin A (30,000 IU twice daily), Vitamin C (500 mg. six times daily).

ULCERS

Ulcers, as they are commonly known, refer to the peptic or gastric (stomach) and duodenal (upper intestine) variety, although they may appear on almost any part of the body, such as bed sores, which are decubitus ulcers. A crater-like lesion is left on the surface of the skin or mucous membrane when dead tissue sloughs off as a result of localized necrosis (tissue death). Gastric juices eat away the lining of the stomach or duodenum causing bleeding in severe situations. This can result in shock, anemia and other complications. A perforated ulcer occurs when the juices eat right through the mucous membrane. Severe inflammation of the peritoneal membrane lining the abdominal cavity may result, accompanied by a substantial amount of persistent pain and often nausea and vomiting.

Recommended Action

Eat smaller but more frequent meals (six to eight light meals daily) to reduce the amount of gastric juices necessary. Thoroughly chewing and salivating each bite will enhance digestion and remove much of the burden from the gastric juices. Unless raw fruits and vegetables are soft, bland kinds such as avocados, bananas and squash, they should be blended, pureed or juiced until recovery is well under way. Avoid citrus and other highly acid fruits for some time and eliminate all fried foods and refined carbohydrates. A specific remedy for duodenal ulcers is raw FRESHLY MADE cabbage juice, while stomach ulcers respond well to raw FRESHLY MADE potato juice. It is important that these remedies be made fresh each time. They may be taken individually, mixed together, or mixed with carrot or celery juices. Drink all liquids (juice, tea and even water) at a temperature as close as possible to that of the body. Cabbage juice often stings the first few times it is taken. A low mucus diet should be adopted. Even though a popular cure for ulcers is to drink plenty of milk, we feel that this will only aggravate the situation in the long run.

Single Herbs: Comfrey (demulcent and cell proliferant), Slippery Elm (soothing and nourishing).

Combinations: Stomach Tonic.

Synergistic Vitamins and Minerals: Calcium/Magnesium (250/125 mg. before meals).

Mucus and Ulcers

We have had great results with ulcers doing just the opposite of the allopaths. We strongly suggest NO Dairy Products or Flour Products. Adopt the Inner cleanse diet for two weeks, pureeing food if necessary. After two weeks remain on the diet but take one Stomach Tonic in the middle of meals.

VAGINAL PROBLEMS

There are a multitude of vaginal problems such as tumors, cysts, polyps, strictures (narrowing or tightening of the tissues), fistulas (abnormal openings from or into another part of the body as a result of injury or infection), hernias (protusions into the vagina by other organs or tissues) and uterine prolapse. Constitutional weakness in the female reproductive organs and supporting structures, which can be complicated by various other factors, is the basic cause of all these problems.

Recommended Action

Emmenagogue herbs have a tonic effect on the muscles and organs of the reproductive area and in combination with other astringent and tissue building herbs can achieve good results in rebuilding and strengthening these tissues. For simple yeast infections the best thing is an acidophilus suppository.

Combinations: Female Formula.

VARICOSE VEINS

Varicose veins usually occur as a result of the valves inside the veins (which normally prevent downward backflow) becoming weakened and failing in their function. This allows blood to fall back down the veinous structure opposite to the normal flow, creating enlarged, twisted and swollen veins. They are commonly found on the legs of older people, pregnant women and those whose occupations require a lot of standing. People who do more walking, or other exercise, are not affected as often because muscular contractions squeeze against the veins to force the blood back up them during exercise. The typical blue varicose veins seen on the surface of the legs are veins which have dilated or expanded as a result of the outward pressure on their walls as abnormal amounts of blood collect in them. The blue color is due to the lack of oxygen in venous blood, which is returning to the heart. Varicosity further disables the valves in the veins, and the situation therefore compounds itself and the veins become grossly distorted along with aching, cramping and general weakness. If sores and ulcers develop, they may be prevented from healing due to inadequate circulation. Thrombophlebitis (severe inflammation of the blood vessels, complicated by blood clots) is a dangerous condition that may then result.

Recommended Action

Much of the weakness of the valves and walls of the veins can be attributed to calcium deficiency, and it should therefore be taken as a supplement. White Oak Bark taken as a tea (simmered down to 1/4 its original amount) or applied as a fomentation is a specific astringent tonic for varicose veins. It can also be painted on like shellac and wrapped with a bandage as well as taken orally.

Single Herbs: White Oak Bark, Collinsonia root.

Combinations: Padma 28, Cleansing Formula.

Synergistic Vitamins and Minerals: Bioflavonoids (1000 mg. three - six times daily), Rutin (500 mg. twice daily), Hesperidin (500 mg. twice daily), Calcium, Multi-Mineral, trace minerals.

WEIGHT CONTROL

Our modern diet and lifestyle makes it virtually impossible to maintain a normal, healthy body weight. Consequently, weight control has become an obsession in our society, but this must necessarily be based on diet control and control over other factors related to optimum health such as exercise, rest, anxiety and stress, boredom, frustration and psychological hunger. Often nutritional deficiencies, metabolic abnormalities and in some cases glandular disorders must first be remedied before weight can be controlled effectively. If parasites are the cause of a voracious appetite, as is often the case, they must be eliminated first. Adopt a diet low in mucus and do periodic juice fasting as well as supplementing with such herbs as are indicated for the specific condition in all the above situations.

Recommended Action

There are so many diet plans on the market that it is ridiculous. In a course at Wild Rose College of Natural Healing, a complete study is made of all the aspects of weight loss, with a lengthy comparison of a number of different programs. We have listed what we consider the best program in the appendix along with the other diets. The reason we feel that the ultimate weight loss program is best is that it considers the metabolic function of the body. This program "tricks" the body into thinking it is fasting but at the same time keeps the metabolism high, thus burning off fat. (Refer to Ultimate Weight Loss Diet in appendix.)

Single Herbs: Oil of Evening Primrose, Chickweed, Glucomannan.

Lymphatic Glands and Weight

Water retention is very common in women and is often the reason for being overweight in later years. Lymphatic problems should be looked after at the youngest possible age. Some young women have signs of lymphatic congestion discovered through Iridology when there is still no sign of water retention. These ladies are usually fairly slender but have mothers who are quite big. You will often find that their mothers were quite slender when they were young too. So if you want to keep a nice figure, look after your lymphatic system.

Combinations: Psyllax .

Synergistic Vitamins and Minerals: Protein powder (predigested if possible), Multi - vitamin and minerals.

APPENDIX

Allergy Testing through Applied Kinesiology

There are many Kinesiology tests that can be used to detect allergies. I use two different types depending on the strength of the person. By testing the strength of various muscles while a person is holding a certain food, cosmetic, cleaning detergent etc. you can often tell if an allergy may be present.

I usually use the shoulder muscle or the finger muscle to test a person for allergies. To start with I test the normal strength of their muscle, as shown in the diagrams. I then get the person to hold the substance being tested in the other hand, close to their stomach if it is considered a 'food'. If the substance is an environmental one, I have the person hold it at half an arm's-length from the body. If the substance has a tendency to cause an allergic reaction it will weaken the muscle tested in either case.

The first few times I did this I couldn't believe it worked, but "the proof of the pudding is in the eating", and after using this method for over seven years I find it quite accurate. The drawback of this method over the Pulse Test is that it only tests the food or substance in its current state. The Pulse Test, however, tests the substance in its state after the body interacts with it. For example a person might not be allergic to potatoes, but due to a poor digestive system, may be allergic to half digested potatoes. The Pulse Test will show this whereas the Kinesiology Test will not.

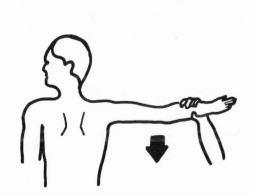

ALLERGY TESTING
THROUGH
SHOULDER MUSCLES

Fig. 1 A

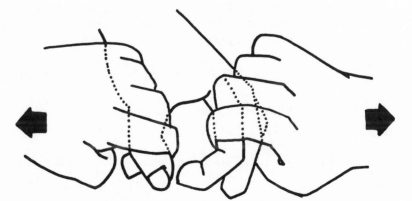

ALLERGY TESTING THROUGH
FINGER MUSCLES

Fig. 1B

Coca's Pulse/Allergy Test

The Pulse Test is another way to test your allergies. It has been noted that the first indication of an allergy is a rise in a person's pulse. By keeping very close watch over the pulse while challenging different foods we can often determine possible allergies. By avoiding foods that cause an increased pulse rate we can aid in clearing allergies and can increase the general health of the person. There are six points to the pulse test.

1. Stop smoking, at least for the duration of the testing, as upon challenging cigarettes they raise the pulse.

2. Take the pulse (usually on the wrist) for ONE WHOLE MINUTE, (not for 1/4 minute and multiplying it by 4, as done in the hospitals) at the following times.
   a) before rising (before sitting up in bed upon waking)
   b) before meals
   c) three times after each meal, at half hour intervals
   d) before retiring for the day

3. Record all foods eaten.

4. Repeat steps 2 and 3 for 2 - 4 days.

5. Do a single food challenge for two or more days. You do this by eating a small portion of a different food every hour, starting early in the morning and continuing for 12 - 14 hours. Take your pulse just before eating the food and one-half hour after.

6. Over the day we have a normal range, one which differs from individual to individual. Any food that seems to elevate the pulse by six (6) points or more should be avoided. These foods should be challenged at other times to see if you get the same results.
   Many allergies involve other than food substances, thereby making the data hard to interpret and resulting in frustration. Some foods do not cause a reaction unless eaten for more than three days in a row. Some allergies do not show up for two or more days after the food is eaten.

Following are some charts to make your task of recording your pulse tests easier.

For more information consult the book:
The Pulse Test
by A.F. Coca M.D.
published by Arco Publishing Company, New York, N.Y.

Chart to test Food Allergies

	Day 1 pulse	Day 2 pulse	Day 3 pulse	Day 4 pulse
Before Rising				
BREAKFAST				
30 min.				
60 min.				
90 min.				
DIET				
LUNCH				
30'				
60'				
90'				
DIET				
DINNER				
30'				
60'				
90'				
DIET				

SINGLE FOOD CHALLENGE

	Day 1 pulse	Day 2 pulse	Day 3 pulse	Day 4 pulse
food				
30 min.				
food				
30'				
food				
30'				
food				
30'				
food				
30'				
food				
30'				
food				
30'				
food				
30'				
food				
30'				
food				
30'				
food				
30'				

ARTHRITIS & RHEUMATISM DIET

No refined grains, sugars, pasta
No salt, baked goods, breads, or processed cereals
No foods containing preservatives
No coffee, black tea
Limited red meats, sweets, dairy products, alcohol
Less than 20% acid-forming foods (see chart)
60% raw food

One tablespoon Norwegian Cod Liver Oil taken straight or in two tablespoons of orange juice or milk, thoroughly shaken, one hour before breakfast. (Nothing else to be taken before breakfast.)

BREAKFAST: One tablespoon apple cider vinegar and 1/2 tablespoon
Unpasteurized honey in 1/2 cup warm water.
Fruit meal - a little yogurt can be added.
It is preferred to have one type of fruit only, e.g. a bowl of cherries and yogurt, or a grapefruit.

Supplements: 500 mg Vitamin C (with bioflavenoids)
Mega B Complex (50 - 60 mg)
1200 mg Lecithin
1 Dulse
2 Cod Liver Oil capsules
2 (Chelated) Bonemeal or
Calcium lactate/Magnesium oxide
2 Multi-minerals with trace minerals
2 Arthritis Formula

Morning Snack: (if desired) Piece of fruit or vegetable, e.g.
carrot sticks or celery or vegetable broth;
cottage cheese or yogurt plus 500 mg Vitamin C
(Vitamin C compulsory)

LUNCH: Major part of meal should be a green salad. Soup or a vegetable can also be eaten.

Supplements: 500 mg Vitamin C
1 Tbsp. Aloe Vera gel containing Irish Moss
2 Arthritis Formula
200 IU Vitamin E

Afternoon Snack: Similar to morning snack.

SUPPER: Big salad, variety of cooked vegetables, a casserole, grain (preferably millet or buckwheat); a little meat can be eaten if desired.

Supplements: Same as for breakfast

Evening Snack: Same as morning snack.

ACID - ALKALINE - ASH CHART

PROTEIN FOODS Column (1) Acid Ash Positive	STARCH FOODS Column (2) Alkaline Ash Negative	BULK FORMING FOODS Column (3) Neutral Starches
Beef	Dates	Asparagus
Pork*	Figs	Celery & Root Celery
Liver	Raisins	Collards
Lamb	Currants	Cabbage
Veal	Maple Syrup	Lettuce
Ham*	Sugar, white/brown*	Beets - Beet tops
Brain	Candy*	Endive
Poultry	Jams - Jellies*	Broccoli
Fish	Cakes - Ice Cream*	Green Peas
Seafoods	Pastries - Pies*	Green Beans
Eggs (whole)	Honey	Water Cress
Yogurt	Molasses	Chives
Buttermilk	Apples	Onions
Wheat Germ	Grapes	Garlic
Rice (white)	Peaches	Mustard
Whole Grains	Pears	Kale
Lentils	Pineapple	Cucumbers
Most nuts (except	Plums	Egg Plant
almonds & brazils)	Melons	Radishes
Natural Cheese	Bananas	Spinach
Cooked Prunes	Cherries	Green Peppers
(no sugar)	Apricots	Okra
Cooked Tomatoes	Cantaloupe	Sorrel
Cooked Rhubarb	Tomatoes (fresh)	Peppermint
Coffee (black)	Pumpkin-Squash	Green Corn
Tea (no sugar)	Potatoes (baked)	Escarole
Soy Beans	Brown Rice	Dandelion
Dried Peas	Millet-Buckwheat	Kohlrabi
Dried Beans	Almonds	Artichokes
	Brazil nuts	Parsley
	Peanuts*	Carrots
	Oily nuts*	Parsnips
	White Flour*	Turnips
	Macaroni*	Rutabagas
	Spaghetti*	Brussel Sprouts
	Cereals (processed)*	Mushrooms
	Flour Gravy*	Avocado
	Popcorn	Butter
	Thick Soups*	Olive Oil
		Cottage cheese

*Those with an asterisk (*) are not recommended at any time.

BREAKING A FAST

A Fast should be broken slowly! It should take half as long to break the fast as the length of the fast (e.g. five days for a ten day fast).

A FOUR-DAY OR LESS FAST

Day One: Eat melons; if unavailable, other juicy fruit, small portions only.

Day Two: Fruit for breakfast; raw vegetable salads for the rest of the day, still with small portions.

Day Three: At least three days of the Inner Cleanse diet at normal portions.

FIVE DAYS AND OVER

Day One: Eat a small portion of melon for breakfast. Drink diluted apple, grape or orange juice during the day and a small portion of melon for dinner.

Day Two: Eat three fruit meals (small portions); drink fruit juice.

Day Three: Fruit for breakfast; raw vegetable salad for the rest of the day. Drink vegetable juice near vegetable meals and fruit juice near fruit meals.

Day Four: Start on Inner Cleanse diet and remember that it takes half as long as your fast to get to normal portions.

COMPLEX CARBOHYDRATE DIET

No sugar, honey, maple syrup or sweetening agent of any type
No baked goods - only two slices of bread daily
No dried fruit - unless soaked overnight and stewed
No bananas, potatoes or pasta
All fruit juice diluted (50% with distilled water preferred)
No food with preservatives
Little salt
No alcohol
No black tea
No coffee

Fruit juice or a piece of fresh fruit 1/2 hour before breakfast (optional)

BREAKFAST: Grain (quality as in numbered order)
1. millet
2. buckwheat
3. rye or rice
4. cornmeal
5. seven grain cereal
6. other grains

All of these are prepared like rice and eaten on the savory side. A tasty suggestion is to add engevita yeast and Dr. Jensen's Vegetable Seasoning plus some butter or oil.

Morning Snack: vegetable sticks, nuts, fruit, yogurt, buttermilk or cottage cheese; and 500 mg. Vitamin C.

LUNCH: The main part of the meal should be a green salad; soup, a sandwich or a vegetable dish can also be eaten.

Afternoon Snack - same as morning.

SUPPER: The Major part of the meal should be a variety of cooked vegetables. A casserole, grains and/or meat can be added if desired. The addition of a salad is desirable.

Evening Snack - same as morning.

DAILY FOOD REGIME

In the Daily Food Regime there are two basic rules that should be followed: variety and food combination.

The food should be as varied as possible. If a person's diet has variety a wide range of vitamins, minerals and other essential nutrients are provided. It is also good to vary the diet according to the season by trying to eat foods that are "in season". In the summer there is abundant fresh fruit and vegetables and this lighter diet feels much better with the hot summer weather. In the winter the diet should be heavier with more grains, proteins, starches, oils and maybe even meat.

A good general diet over a period of a day would contain two different fruits, at least 4 to 6 vegetables, 1 protein and 1 starch, with fruit or vegetable juice between meals if desired. Eat at least two types of leafy green vegetables daily.

One half hour before breakfast drink unsweetened juice. It is good to follow this with at least 12 minutes of aerobic exercise (if not done at this time it should be done some other time during the day).

BREAKFAST

A fruit with a health drink; a grain with a health drink or a protein with a health drink.

LUNCH (Lunch and Dinner may be interchanged)

Raw salad, one starch and a health drink.

DINNER (Lunch and Dinner may be interchanged)

A small raw salad, at least two cooked vegetables, one protein, and a broth or health drink if desired.

GRAINS: Millet, buckwheat, cornmeal, rice, barley, seven grain cereal, Red River cereal, Roman Meal.

PROTEIN: If vegetarian: Beans, (preferably sprouted and/or slow cooked) nut butters, tofu, curded dairy (if desired) and high protein vegetables.
If you eat meat: Fish or poultry twice a week, lean meat twice a week, curded dairy once a week, eggs once a week (preferably soft, poached or boiled).

VEGETABLES: Artichokes, asparagus, beans, beets, broccoli, brussel sprouts, cabbage, carrots, cauliflower, cucumber, celery, dandelion, endive, corn, peas, peppers, kale, kohlrabi, lettuce, lotus, okra, sprouts, onions, garlic, parsley, parsnips, pumpkin, radishes, rutabagas, salsify, spinach, squash, swiss chard, turnip, zucchini, tomatoes, avocado, and eggplant.

STARCHES: Baked potato or grain.

HEALTH DRINK: Vegetable broth, coffee substitute, curded dairy blender drink, herbal tea. Many people feel it is good to have three to seven favourite herbal drinks, rotating them for variety, in a cycle. Some good teas for this are oatstraw, comfrey, alfamint, parsley, raspberry, grain tea and dandelion root tea.

FOOD NOTES:

You should never eat protein and starches or proteins and sweets together. You may wish to trade the evening and noon meals around. It takes exercise to handle raw food and we generally get more exercise after our noon meal. Starches also need exercise so if one eats sandwiches, the time to do so is usually at noon. Fruit can be substituted for any of these meals. If you do not feel hungry or do not feel well, a fruit meal is often the best food to eat.

RULES OF EATING

1. If you are not comfortable in mind and body (in pain, emotionally upset, not hungry, chilled, overheated, during acute illness) you should miss the meal.
2. Be sure to chew your food thoroughly.
3. Do not eat beyond your needs.

THREE-DAY DETOXIFICATION DIET

This three-day detoxification fast has done wonders for many people, eliminating mucus, chemical and drug deposits, while helping to revitalize the body. (Times given may be varied to suit your schedule, as long as the intervals are maintained).

DAY ONE
On arising drink eight ounces of prune juice. In 1/2 hour drink another eight ounces of prune juice. The rest of the day drink as much apple juice as possible, diluted 50/50 with distilled water, until 6:00 P.M.

Take nothing between 6:00 and 9:00 p.m. At 9:00 make and drink the following mixture:
>   juice of two oranges
>   juice of one lemon
>   5 - 10 tablespoons olive oil
>   1 - 3 cloves of garlic (if desired) finely chopped
>   Blend in a blender or shake thoroughly.
>   Take nothing else until 8:00 a.m. the next morning.

DAY TWO
Do a warm water enema. Drink eight ounces of prune juice. Start drinking diluted apple juice and repeat day one.

DAY THREE
Repeat day two.

Do not take any vitamins or other supplements during this period unless otherwise stated. Take 2 Lower Bowel Tonic three times daily.

The more apple juice you drink, the more cleansing is accomplished.

REMEMBER, DRINK SLOWLY!

INNER CLEANSE DIET

If you are preceding the Inner Cleanse with the Detoxification Diet, eat small quantities of raw food on the first day, building up to start the full Inner Cleanse diet over a period half as long as your fast, (e.g. for a 10 day fast, take 5 days to reach full proportions).

For the Inner Cleanse diet you will be able to FEAST - not fast! The idea is to fill your body with natural precious vitamins and minerals. When a sufficient amount of these live substances reaches the cells of your body, there will be a cleansing and elimination of toxic material throughout it. This program will be a good start for you to have a strong, healthy body with lots of energy. Follow the directions carefully.

NO dairy products (except where noted), potatoes (yams are OK), avocadoes
NO dried fruit, grains, beans
NO tomatoes, baked goods (except where noted), eggplant
NO sugar, honey, maple syrup or sweetening agent of any type
NO bananas, pasta, preserved food, meat
NO coffee, black tea, or alcohol
Little salt
Stop all supplements for duration of Cleanse unless otherwise specified.

BEFORE BREAKFAST

Fifteen minutes before you are ready to eat breakfast, squeeze the juice of a lemon in a medium glass of hot water and drink it.

BREAKFAST

APPLE OR GRAPEFRUIT JUICE - eight ounces minimum. You can take more if you desire, but be sure that you take at least eight ounces.
YOGURT - up to five tablespoons of plain yogurt (if desired)
FRESH FRUIT - one-half pound. You may eat more, but be sure to eat at least one-half pound.
(REMEMBER: NO BANANAS OR AVOCADOES)

LUNCH

VEGETABLE MINERAL BROTH - Drink two cups during the meal.
SALAD - Make a chopped salad of fresh raw vegetables. Use a dressing of olive oil, lemon juice, kelp or dulse and engevita yeast (if desired). Eat at least eight level tablespoonsful of salad. Use at least four of the following vegetables: artichokes, asparagus, beans, beets, broccoli, brussel sprouts, cabbage, carrots cauliflower, cucumber, celery, dandelion, endive, corn, peas, peppers, kale, kohlrabi, lettuce, lotus, okra, sprouts, onions, garlic, parsley, parsnips, pumpkin, radishes, rutabaga, salsify, spinach, squash, swiss chard, turnip, zucchini.

DINNER

VEGETABLE MINERAL BROTH - Drink two cups during the meal.

COOKED VEGETABLES - Select three or more of the vegetables listed for lunch and steam or stir fry them in butter. Eat a generous portion. Cooked vegetables are necessary in the evening for proper cleansing. A salad can be added.

BREAD - One medium slice of whole grain bread with butter (if desired).

SNACKS - Between meals you should drink all the fruit or vegetable juice you like. You may also eat raw vegetables or fruits. You should allow at least 1/2 hour between eating fruit and eating vegetables. The more live food you can eat or drink, the more cleansing will be done. If fresh fruit juice cannot be obtained, canned varieties from the Health Food store will do. Make the Vegetable Mineral Broth and drink as much as you like.

VEGETABLE MINERAL BROTH

2 cups carrot tops (leaves)
2 cups potato peels, 1/4 inch thick
2 cups beet tops
3 cups celery (stalks and leaves)
2 cups parsley (1 cup dehydrated)

Cover with distilled water and simmer for 20 minutes. Strain, keep broth and discard vegetables. If one of the vegetables is unobtainable, just leave it out. (Replace it with one of the other vegetables if possible.)

You can add garlic, onion or other vegetables and vegetable ends. Some people like to add miso, soya sauce or Dr. Jensen's "Vegetable Broth or Seasoning" in the last few minutes for taste.

Drink hot or cold.

If time is limited you can take one tablespoon of Dr. Jensen's "Vegetable Broth or Seasoning" and pour one cup of boiled water over it as a substitute.

"LEMON AID" CLEANSE

The "Lemon Aid" Cleanse is designed for eliminating toxins and congestion while revitalizing the body. We use this cleanse in some of the longer cleansing programs, for it doesn't create a lack of physical energy even after ten days. In its simplicity it is easy to follow at home, at work or while travelling. The major part of the cleanse is drinking the following mixture:

2 tablespoons of freshly squeezed lemons or limes
1 tablespoon Maple Syrup
1/10 teaspoon Cayenne pepper (more if desired)

Take this mixture and put it in 8 - 10 ounces of water, warm or cold. The lemons or limes have to be fresh, not canned; organic ones are best if possible. The Maple Syrup should be grade B or C, as they are higher in mineral content.

We have found it is sometimes more convenient to make up a day's supply at one time. We do this with:

2 cups freshly squeezed lemons
1 cup Maple Syrup
1 or more teaspoons of Cayenne

Of this mixture, take three tablespoonsful per 8 - 10 ounce glass.

You should drink between 6 and 12 glasses daily (more if desired). If you also want to lose weight with this program, keep close to six cups daily.

During this cleansing we have to keep the bowel active (to eliminate toxins), so for the first three mornings do an enema with warm water. We also suggest:
2 Lower Bowel Tonic, 3 times daily (increase if necessary)

During the cleanse, take no vitamins or other supplements unless otherwise specified. Of course **no** food is taken during this period. For a change, you could drink a cup of mint tea in the evening.

REMEMBER: DRINK SLOWLY!

LIVER FLUSH

The Liver Flush is a wholesale cleansing of the body and should only be done under a practitioner's care.

This Liver Flush is best preceded with one month of liver herbs such as Liver Formula (two capsules - three times daily) and/or the three day detoxification fast.

In the morning do an enema or colonic; one half-hour later drink eight ounces of prune juice. Drink diluted apple juice only (mixed half and half with distilled water) until 6:00 p.m. Don't take in anything until 9:00 p.m. At that time measure out:

1 - 1 1/2 cups pure olive oil (cold pressed)
1 - 1 1/2 cups freshly squeezed lemon juice

Take three tablespoons of each; wait 15 minutes and repeat until finished (about three hours). Try not to stop even if you become nauseated or vomit. Try to continue until you are finished, as you are performing a thorough cleansing of toxins and mucus.

When you are ready to go to bed, sleep on your right side, to put slight pressure on the liver.

If you wake up very nauseated and feel you can't go on, and **ONLY** if you can't go on, take one tablespoon of pure gelatin, rinse your mouth with water and go back to sleep. This will completely stop the action of the cleanse.

In the morning do two enemas or preferably have a colonic.

THE ULTIMATE WEIGHT LOSS PROGRAM

This weight loss program doesn't just help you lose weight that you will gain back a week later. This is a program which aids in adjusting the "idle" of your metabolic rate. Your body will start to burn up fat, changing weight into muscle, thereby not only reducing bulk but making you more shapely. So let's start with shaping up and keeping fit!

BREAKFAST
2 Tablespoons of Psyllax (in a liquid)
2 Tablespoons of Protein Powder (in a liquid)
1 Multiple Vitamin/Mineral

LUNCH
1 Tablespoon Psyllax
2 Tablespoons Protein Powder
1 Multiple Vitamin/Mineral

Eat a bowl of clear vegetable soup made from non-starchy vegetables.

SUPPER
2 Tablespoons Psyllax
2 Tablespoons Protein Powder
1 Multiple Vitamin/Mineral

Eat a salad of non-starchy vegetables.

Lunch and Supper can be exchanged.

Drink at least 12 cups of fluid during the day. The Psyllax tastes best in Tomato Juice. Any liquid may be used with the Protein Powder.

Do at least 15 minutes of aerobic exercise daily.

The diet must be done for more than five days to be effective and not more than twenty days followed by a ten-day break, and repeated if desired.

QUESTIONS AND ANSWERS

SHOULD VITAMINS AND MINERALS BE USED TOGETHER WITH HERBS?

I feel that vitamins, minerals, herbs, diet, exercise, and mental and emotional attitudes are all part of a wholistic healing program and cannot be separated. If you were building a brick house, you might want a forklift or bulldozer to help you lift the bricks into place. In building this foundation we can liken the bricks to minerals as they are building blocks of the body. Vitamins are similar to the gasoline used to run the bulldozer (Vitamins often work as co-enzymes to activate enzymes) and the bulldozer itself is like the body's enzymes that catalyze actions in the body. Now, we **could** build a house with these few substances, but a simple house it would be! If we were then to add herbs (which also contain vitamins, minerals, enzymes and other substances) to our own building program, it would be similar to adding a foreman to the construction project. Now we can create a house with a few fancy trimmings! Because of the cleansing nature of herbs we are even left with some workers to clean and tidy up the mess after the building is complete.

Many would say at this point, "If herbs are so good, why not use them alone?" Herbs, like vitamins and minerals, may be used alone. The best and fastest results, however, are obtained when all of the raw materials for the construction are already in the form required for that construction. By using all three together you have all the parts present right at the start of the building, without having to spend time and energy recycling used parts to get the other raw materials needed. This is especially important because some of those "used parts", which were recycled are used later in the building process in their original form!

So, not only should we combine vitamins, minerals and herbs, we should be careful to include exercise, diet, and mental/emotional attitudes in our building process.

HOW MANY HERBAL FORMULAS SHOULD A PERSON USE AT THE SAME TIME?

In general, I would say that a person should not be working on more than four areas of the body at one time. (Of course, as with every rule, there are exceptions.) However, this does not directly answer the question, as a woman may be working on one area, female organs for example, but will be using a Female Corrective formula, a Dong Quai formula and Vitamin E. This constitutes only one problem area, and the woman may work on up to three other organs or tissues at the same time. The number of **formulas** then depends on the nature of the individual problems.

ARE THERE ANY HERBAL FORMULAS THAT SHOULD NOT BE USED WITH OTHER HERBAL FORMULAS?

Specific information as to the combinations involved would provide the most accurate answer. As with medical drugs, certain herbs do not combine well, and it is a general practice not to work on diverse areas of the body at exactly the same time. If you were working on the heart and the colon, the best results would be obtained by taking the formulas at different times of day, say at breakfast and lunch. If you try to work on two areas at the same time, the vital energies of the body are pulled in two different directions, giving less power for healing in both areas. If, however, you were dealing with the pancreas, liver and large intestine, then there is a vast difference: all are related to the digestive system so the energy being applied is kept localized.

HOW LONG DOES ONE HAVE TO USE HERBS RELATIVE TO VITAMINS?

When using herbal formulas we are dealing with a more definite time period than for the use of vitamins. If a formula were being used for kidneys, we would continue use until the organ built up its strength, usually a period of three to nine months (more in some cases). Vitamins, though, are chemicals necessary for life support that are not produced in the body in sufficient quantity to maintain it. Because of this vitamins must be consumed regularly throughout our lives either in our diet or in pill form. Many of these vitamin needs can be supplied from our diet, but the vitamin content of the foods we eat is deteriorating and the stress of the modern world is placing a larger vitamin demand on us. This is where vitamin supplements may make the difference.

Herbs are used as a relatively short-term tool and the need for them lasts only as long as the problem exists. Once the healing is done, and as long as we keep from the habits that gave us the problems in the first place, the herbs may no longer be needed.

WHERE SHOULD I START IF I WANT TO GO ON A HERBAL PROGRAM?

Each health program is highly individualized, but it is usual to begin at the digestive system. If this system is not working adequately, there will be inefficient absorption of the nutrients, herbs and vitamins that are taken to help other systems and organs of the body.

WHAT WOULD BE A STEP-BY-STEP PROGRAM FOR BUILDING UP THE BODY?

After cleaning the digestive system to permit more efficient use of the nutrients supplied, we usually move to work on the eliminatory organs: colon, kidneys, lungs and skin. With these systems operating well we can remove toxin buildup inside the body. At this time, too, we can start to build the other specific vital areas of the individual that require attention. These would include the heart, liver, endocrine glands and nervous system. From this point we would start to concentrate on less vital areas.

WHAT IS A HEALING CRISIS?

The concept of the Healing Crisis is found in a Homeopathic Law called Hering's Law of Cure, which states that all cure comes from within out, from the head down and in the reverse order of the appearance of the symptoms.

Let us take the example of a person who goes to a drugstore upon "catching" a cold. The product purchased is one advertised to relieve the symptoms of a cold. This product will likely relieve the symptoms of the cold, but it probably won't do much more that is beneficial. It will, in all likelihood, dry up and crystallize the mucus and toxins being released through the action of the cold, driving them deeply into the bronchial tissues. This changes the condition from acute to subacute, a less noticeable state, making the person feel better. Some time later (often at the change of a season) the body will make its attempt to throw these toxins off. This may result in a cold, cough or even the flu, which frequently drives the person back to the time-tested formula used earlier to relieve the "problem". This, of course, reverses the cleansing at once, driving the mucus and toxins ever more deeply into the tissues. Starting with a cold, a usual history is to develop tendencies to coughs, flus, bronchitis or hayfever, then asthma and finally, perhaps, a degenerate and chronically diseased lung.

At some stage, however, the person may decide to begin living in a more healthy manner and eventually begins to feel better. This healthy period progresses happily until the person is usually heard to remark, "I haven't felt this good in years!". At this point the body has built up enough strength again so that it attempts once more to eliminate some of the toxins. In our example the person might appear to "catch" asthma, which he hasn't had for years. During this crisis, the body is simply trying to rid itself of the toxins and the disharmonies.

Throughout a cleansing/building program there will be periods of better health punctuated by short crises. The person in our example will then, over perhaps months or years, re-experience asthma, hayfever, bronchitis, flus, coughs and colds, in that order. Each of these conditions will appear as a Healing Crisis, with symptoms similar to that of the original disease crisis. The major difference is that the crisis is of much shorter duration and is often more dramatic. The person also feels much better both before and after the crisis (if left to run its natural course). The individual should ensure the intake of plenty of vitamins, minerals, herbs specific to the problem and brothy soups to promote a speedy recovery.

GLOSSARY OF HERBAL TERMS

Alterative	Producing a healthful change without perception.
Anodyne	Relieves mild pain.
Anthelmintic	A medicine that expels worms.
Antibilious	Acts on the bile, relieving biliousness.
Antiemetic	Stops vomiting.
Antiperiodic	Preventing regular recurrences.
Antilithic	Prevents the formation of stones in the urinary organs.
Antirheumatic	Relieves or cures rheumatism.
Antiscorbutic	Cures or prevents scurvy.
Antiseptic	A medicine that prevents putrefaction.
Antispasmodic	Relieves or prevents spasms.
Antisyphilitic	Having effect of curing or relieving syphilis.
Aperient	Gently laxative without purging.
Aromatic	A stimulant, spicy, anti-griping.
Astringent	Causes contraction and arrests discharges.
Carminative	Expels wind from the bowels.
Cathartic	Evacuates the bowels, (a purgative).
Cephalic	Pertaining to the head.
Cholagogue	Increases the flow of bile into the intestine.
Condiment	Improves the flavour of foods.
Demulcent	Soothing, relieves inflammation, especially for skin and mucous membranes.
Deobstruent	Removes obstruction.
Depurative	Purifies the blood.
Detergent	Cleansing.
Diaphoretic	Produces perspiration.
Discutient	Dissolves and heals tumours.
Diuretic	Increases the secretion and flow of urine.
Emetic	Produces vomiting.
Emmenagogue	Promotes menstruation.
Emollient	Softens and soothes inflamed parts when locally applied.
Esculent	Edible.
Exanthematous	Pertaining to skin eruptions and diseases.
Expectorant	Facilitates expulsion of mucus or phlegm from the lungs and throat.
Febrifuge	Abates and reduces fevers.
Hepatic	Pertaining to the liver.
Laxative	Promotes bowel action.
Lithotriptic	Dissolves calculi (stones) in the urinary organs.
Mucilaginous	Soothing to all inflammations.
Nauseant	Produces vomiting.
Nervine	Acts specifically on the nervous system, stops nervous excitement, tonic.
Parturient	Induces and promotes labour at childbirth.
Pectoral	A remedy for chest afflictions.

Refrigerant	Cooling.
Resolvent	Dissolves boils, tumours, and other inflammations.
Rubefacient	Increases circulation and produces red skin.
Sedative	Quiets nerve action and promotes sleep.
Sialogogue	Increases the secretion of saliva.
Stomachic	Excites the action of the stomach, has the effect of strengthening it and relieving indigestion.
Styptic	Arrests hemorrhage.
Sudorific	Produces profuse perspiration.
Tonic	A remedy which is invigorating, strengthening, and toning.
Vermifuge	Expels worms from the intestines.

INDEX

Recommended Readings

Herbals

A Modern Herbal by M. Grieve; Penguin, Middlesex, England; 1931
School of Natural Healing by Dr. J. R. Christopher; BiWorld Publishers, Provo Utah; 1976
Green Pharmacy B. Griggs; Jill Norman & Hobhouse Ltd., London, Eng; 1981
The Way of Herbs; M. Tierra; Orenda/Unity Press, Santa Cruz; 1980
Herbal Medication: A Clinical and Depensary Handbook;A.W. Priest and L.R. Priest; L. N. Fowler & Co. Ltd, London,Eng.; 1982
Indian Herbology; A. Hutchens; Merco, Windsor Ont. Canada; 1969
The Herb Book; J. Lust; Bantam Books, New York; 1974

Advanced Herbology

Encyclopedia of Common Natural Ingredients Used in Food, Drugs and Cosmetics; A. Y. Leung; John Wiley and Son, New York; 1980
Herbal Medications; D. G. Spoerke; Woodbridge Press Publishing Co., Santa Barbara; 1980
The Organic Constituents of Higher Plants; Fourth edition; T. Robinson; University of Massachusetts, Amherst Mass; 1980

Nutrition/Vitamins

The Nutrition Desk Reference; R. Garrison & E. Somer; Keating Publishing, New Canaan, Connecticut; 1985.
How To Get Well; P. Airola; Health Plus Publishers, Phoenix Arizona; 1974.
Nutraerobics; J. Bland; Harper & Row, San Francisco; 1983.
The Pulse Test; A. Coca; Arc Books, New York; 1956.
Comprehensive answer to Nutrition; W. Borrman; New Horizons, Chicago; 1979.
Vitamin Bible; E. Mindell; Warner Books; New York; 1985.
Modern Nutrition in Health and Disease (Sixth Edition); R.S. Goodhart & M.E. Shils; Lea & Febiger, Philadelphia; 1980.

Author's Availability for Lectures

Terry Willard, Ph.D. is one of North America's most sought after natural health speakers and herbal consultants. His formulas have been used by North Americans and Europeans for close to a decade. A commitment to the development of health routines based on the best of tradition and science have placed him in a position of leadership in the renaissance of natural remedies.

While he spends a great deal of his time in his Calgary clinic he is available for personal appearances and consulting to a certain degree.

For more information please contact:

Research Co-ordinator
Chiron Consulting
302, 1220 Kensington Rd. N.W.
Calgary, Alberta, CANADA
T2N 3P5
(403) 270-7110

Wild Rose College of Natural Healing

The Wild Rose College of Natural Healing Ltd. has been giving both classroom and correspondence instruction in many areas of health since the mid-70's. With active correspondence students from all parts of the globe, the College provides a source of knowledge to those who cannot travel to the few institutions of advanced learning in natural healing.

The College offers two diplomas: Master Herbalist (M.H.) and Wholistic Therapist (W.T.). Full-time study for the period of one year usually permits completion of a degree.

For further information, please send $3.00 for a College calendar to:

College Co-ordinator
Wild Rose College of Natural Healing, Ltd.
302, 1220 Kensington Rd. N.W.
Calgary, Alberta, CANADA
T2N 3P5
(403) 270-0936

Other Herbal Manuals

TWO NEW BOOKS BY TERRY WILLARD, PH.D.:
Available Fall, 1986 from Wild Rose College
(address on previous page)

TEXTBOOK OF MODERN HERBOLOGY....hardcover, approx. 350 pages

Based on the highly praised introductory herbology course of the Wild Rose College of Natural Healing, the **Textbook** gives a thorough grounding in physiology and herbology. Useful as a first textbook of herbal study, the information on botany, human anatomy and biochemistry reflects the most modern form of North American herbology practised today. Major categories of herbs are included, making the **Textbook of Modern Herbology** a must for the bookshelf of serious students and practitioners of Western herbology.

THE WILD ROSE SCIENTIFIC HERBAL....hardcover, approx. 250 pages

The result of ten years of research and compilation by Terry Willarad, Ph.D., the **Scientific Herbal** promises to take the field of herbology into a new scientific era. Over 200 herbs are reviewed for their biochemical effects. Dosage levels, toxicity, common names and folklore are all covered with academic citation standards. The reference list is extensive and includes other modern scientific bibliographies on herbs. Volumes similar to the **Scientific Herbal** all cost three to four times as much and do not have the advantage of being assembled by a practising herbalist. **The Wild Rose Scientific Herbal** will be the desk reference for any natural health practitioner, pharmacist or medical doctor with an interest in the facts about herbs.

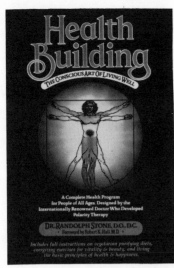

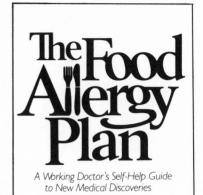

HEALTH BOOKS FROM CRCS PUBLICATIONS

HEALTH BUILDING: The Conscious Art of Living Well by Dr. Randolph Stone, D.C., D.O. 190 pages, paperback $7.95. A complete health regimen for people of all ages by an internationally renowned doctor who specialized in problem cases. Includes instructions for vegetarian purifying diets and energizing exercises for vitality and beauty. Illustrated with drawings & photographs.

TAI CHI: TEN MINUTES TO HEALTH by Chia Siew Pang & Dr. Goh Ewe Hock 8 x 10 **sewn** paperback, over 600 photographs and illustrations...................$12.95 The most comprehensive manual on Yang style Tai Chi available, which breaks down the movements in more detail than any other book. Recommended by American Library Association's Booklist.

HELPING YOURSELF WITH NATURAL REMEDIES: An Encyclopedic Guide to Herbal & Nutritional Treatment by Terry Willard, Ph.D....144-page paperback. This easily accessible book blends 20th Century scientific & clinical experience with traditional methods of health maintenance. Allows reader to select natural remedies for over 100 specific problems, all arranged in alphabetical order & with a complete index!............................$8.95

POLARITY THERAPY: The Complete Collected Works by the Founder of the System Dr. Randolph Stone, D.O.,D.C. (In 2 volumes, 8½ x 11), $25.00 per volume. The original books on this revolutionary healing art available for the first time in trade editions. Fully illustrated with charts & diagrams. Sewn paperbacks, over 500 total pages. Enlightening for students of all the healing arts.

THE FOOD ALLERGY PLAN: A Working Doctor's Self-Help Guide to New Medical Discoveries by Dr. Keith Mumby...210 pages....................................$5.95 Currently a best-seller in England, this book provides the most up-to-date information on guiding the reader in discovering the hidden food allergies affecting perhaps half the population that cause a myriad of psychological and physical problems. Clearly written & easy to use, this book also explains Candida symptoms, effects of pollution, use of supplements, etc..

YOGA FOR THE WEST: A Manual for Designing Your Own Practice by Ian Rawlinson.........................$12.95 A large-size, profusely illustrated paperback with a sewn binding that opens flat for easy use, this pioneering book provides for the Western student of yoga what they have long known they needed--a guide to adapting the ancient principles to the modern person's needs without sacrificing the essence of traditional yoga.

CHINESE VEGETARIAN COOKERY by Jack Santa Maria...6 x 9 paperback...$7.95 Vegetarian magazine called this "the best" of all the books on Chinese vegetarian cookery. It is by far the most accessible for Westerners and uses ingredients that are easily found anywhere. A beautiful, full-color cover (featuring a Chinese painting from the British Museum) sets off this attractive book that all vegetarians and lovers of Chinese food will want to own.